# Kaizen to Pilates and Beyond

## Illustrated

### Karin van der Westhuizen

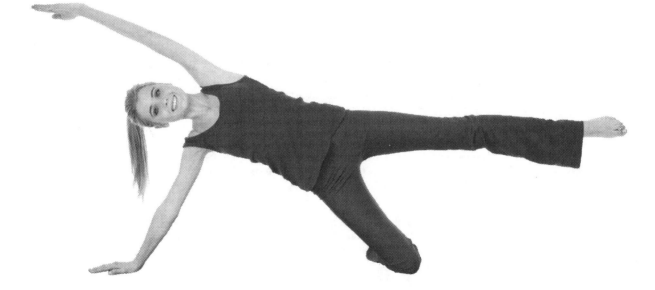

*Kaizen a Japanese word for Continuous Improvement*

**BALBOA**
PRESS
A DIVISION OF HAY HOUSE

Balboa Press books may be ordered through booksellers or by contacting:

Balboa Press
A Division of Hay House
1663 Liberty Drive
Bloomington, IN 47403
www.balboapress.com
1 (877) 407-4847

Because of the dynamic nature of the Internet, any web addresses or links contained in this book may have changed since publication and may no longer be valid. The views expressed in this work are solely those of the author and do not necessarily reflect the views of the publisher, and the publisher hereby disclaims any responsibility for them.

The author of this book does not dispense medical advice or prescribe the use of any technique as a form of treatment for physical, emotional, or medical problems without the advice of a physician, either directly or indirectly. The intent of the author is only to offer information of a general nature to help you in your quest for emotional and spiritual well-being. In the event you use any of the information in this book for yourself, which is your constitutional right, the author and the publisher assume no responsibility for your actions.

Any people depicted in stock imagery provided by Thinkstock are models, and such images are being used for illustrative purposes only.
Certain stock imagery © Thinkstock.

ISBN: 978-1-4525-9113-1 (sc)
ISBN: 978-1-4525-9114-8 (e)

Printed in the United States of America.

Balboa Press rev. date: 11/20/2014

# Contents

# Introduction

## Purpose

The main purpose of Kaizen to Pilates and Beyond *is to provide a good assortment of interesting Pilates and Stretch exercises using a variety of props. The exercises are designed for beginners through to advanced levels of fitness and for trainers to use as a reference.*

*There are more than 150 Pilates exercises and 100 Stretch exercises.*

## Practical manual

*There are easily understandable descriptions and specially choreographed illustrations for each exercise. Above all, this is a practical manual that can help towards achieving and maintaining a good level of fitness.*

## Disclaimer

*Every effort has been made to assemble a set of safe and well tried instructions, however as you will be aware, all exercise involves risk. The risk you take is your responsibility.*

*Consult your doctor before trying these exercises as they are not intended to replace the advice of a medical professional.*

## Accreditations

*Photographs by* Matt Geeling

*Models* Nadia Herbst *and* Carle Latsky

*Editing by* Romy Sacks

*Everything that could have been said about exercises*

*has already been said in so many ways,*

*so now ...*

# *Let's just do it!!!*

---

## *The six principles of the Pilates Movement*

**1** *Concentration*

Concentrate on your exercise and do it with full commitment.

**2** *Control*

Do every Pilates exercise with complete muscular control.

**3** *Centring*

Focus on your core strength stabilisation which is your powerhouse.
Every exercise starts from a strong centre.

**4** *Flowing movement*

Allow your body to flow into the movement.

**5** *Precision*

Pay attention to every detail of every exercise.
This ensures your body is working in the correct manner.

**6** *Breathing*

Breathing is an integral part of Pilates exercises.
Co-ordinate your breathing to the exercises.

---

# Pilates

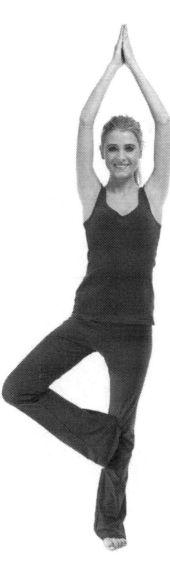

*Pilates develops the body uniformly,
corrects wrong postures,
restores physical vitality,
invigorates the mind
and elevates the spirit*

Joseph Pilates

## *Why do we need to exercise?*

The most important reason of all, the heart, being a muscle, needs exercise to function efficiently. Exercising the heart gives us better blood circulation, which results in …

- ✓ Increased energy

- ✓ Increased metabolism

- ✓ Increased muscle tone

- ✓ Better health

- ✓ Reduced stress

- ✓ Improved self esteem

# Warming Up

*A good warm up is essential to any workout and reduces the risk of injuries. When you do your warming up exercises you raise your body temperature and warm up your muscles and joints and therefore you prepare your body for the more strenuous exercises that follow.*

*Breathing is an essential part of Pilates exercises. Breathe in to feel your ribcage expanding and breathe out to engage into the abdominals. Co-ordinate your exercises by inhaling as you prepare and exhaling as you execute your exercise.*

*Lazy breathing converts the lungs literally and figuratively speaking into a cemetery for the deposition of diseased, dying and dead germs as well as supplying an ideal haven for the multiplication of other harmful germs.*

*Joseph Pilates*

## Pectoral stretch

| | |
|---|---|
| **Setup** | Standing with feet hip-width apart, hands at back on hips, fingers facing down |
| **Exhale** | Push elbows away from body, expand your chest (feel as if someone is pulling your elbows away from your body) |
| **Inhale** | Relax |
| | Repeat 6 x |

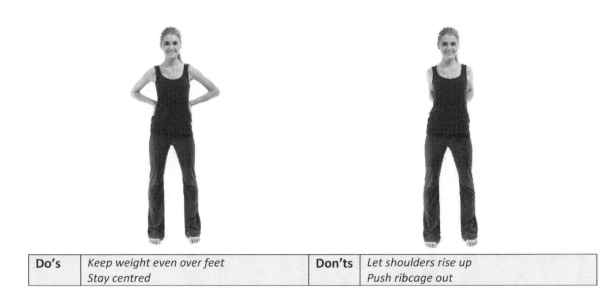

| Do's | Keep weight even over feet<br>Stay centred | Don'ts | Let shoulders rise up<br>Push ribcage out |
|---|---|---|---|

## Forward lunge

**Setup**    Standing with left leg in front, point toe at back, front foot slightly turned out for balance
**Exhale**   Bend front knee, push heel of back foot into floor, leg straight
**Inhale**   Stretch both legs
             Repeat 5 x change legs and repeat

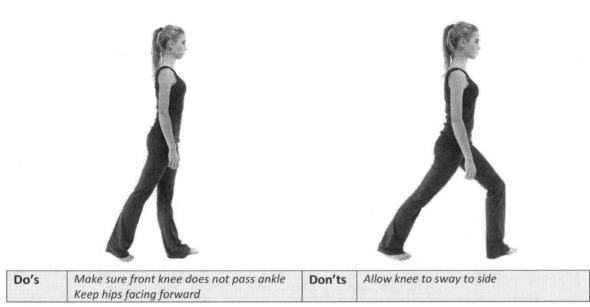

| Do's | Make sure front knee does not pass ankle<br>Keep hips facing forward | Don'ts | Allow knee to sway to side |
| --- | --- | --- | --- |

## Backward lunge

**Setup**    Standing with left leg in front, both knees bent, front foot slightly turned out for balance
**Exhale**   Straighten back leg, push your heel away from your body
**Inhale**   Bend back leg
             Repeat 5 x change legs and repeat

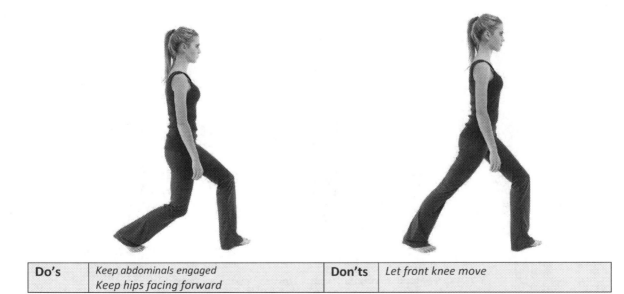

| Do's | Keep abdominals engaged<br>Keep hips facing forward | Don'ts | Let front knee move |
| --- | --- | --- | --- |

## Forward lunge with back extensions

**Setup**      Standing with left leg in front, knee bent, foot slightly turned out for balance
**Exhale**     Lift arms in line with your ears and lean forward into 45 degree angle
**Inhale**      Body upright and arms down to sides
               Repeat 5 x change legs and repeat

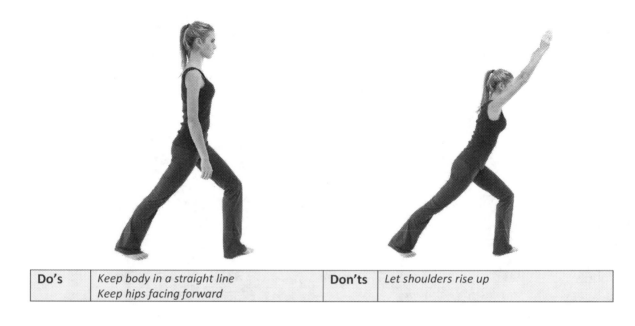

| Do's | Keep body in a straight line<br>Keep hips facing forward | Don'ts | Let shoulders rise up |
|------|-----------------------------------|--------|-----------------------|

## Front and back leg lift

**Setup**      Standing with one foot slightly forward, both knees bent, weight on back leg
**Exhale**     Lift front foot just off the floor
**Inhale**      Step on front foot
               Lift back foot off floor
               Repeat 5 x change legs and repeat

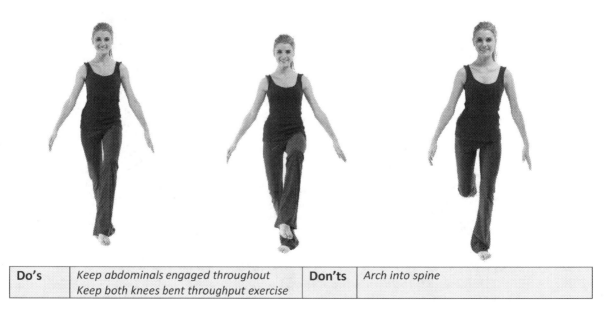

| Do's | Keep abdominals engaged throughout<br>Keep both knees bent throughput exercise | Don'ts | Arch into spine |
|------|-----------------------------------|--------|-----------------|

## Sideways balance

**Setup**     Point right foot to side and stretch left arm
**Exhale**    Lift right leg to side and lean to left side
**Inhale**     Lower leg to floor and repeat to opposite side
            Repeat 10 x alternating sides

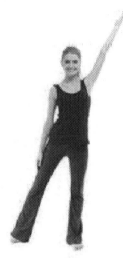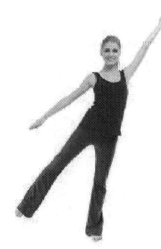

| Do's | Keep abdominals engaged throughout<br>Lengthen out between arm and leg | Don'ts | Sink into supporting leg |
|------|------|------|------|

## Reaching forward balance

**Setup**     Point right foot at back, stretch arms forward
**Exhale**    Lean forward, lift arms in line with ears, lift your leg at the back
**Inhale**     Straighten body and point left foot at back
            Repeat 10 x alternating sides

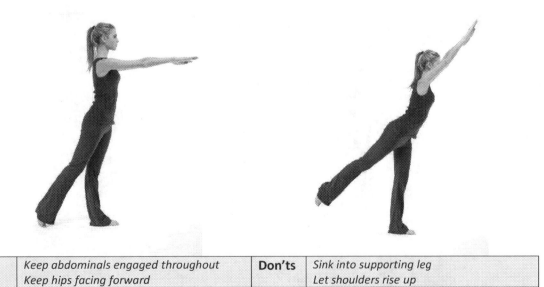

| Do's | Keep abdominals engaged throughout<br>Keep hips facing forward | Don'ts | Sink into supporting leg<br>Let shoulders rise up |
|------|------|------|------|

## Standing leg circles

**Setup**   Standing with feet together, arms to sides
**Inhale**   Stretch leg to front
**Exhale**   Circle leg to the back
**Inhale**   Feet together
Repeat 10 x alternating sides

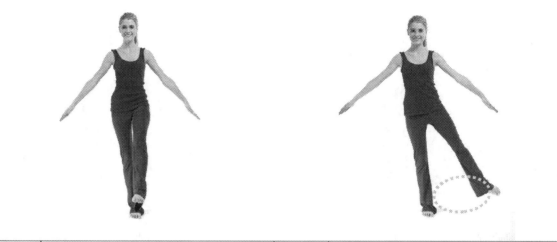

| Do's | Keep abdominals engaged<br>Keep weight centred | Don'ts | Sink into supporting leg<br>Let hips sway backwards or forwards |
|------|------|------|------|

## Balance with stretch

**Setup**   Standing with feet together, arms to sides
**Inhale**   Stretch leg out to side and lift arms shoulder level
**Exhale**   Bend leg and place foot against knee, stretch arms palms together
**Inhale**   Lower leg, bring feet together
Repeat 10 x alternating sides

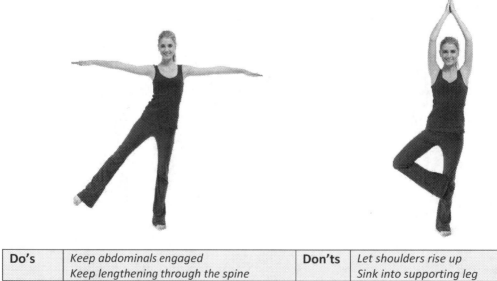

| Do's | Keep abdominals engaged<br>Keep lengthening through the spine | Don'ts | Let shoulders rise up<br>Sink into supporting leg |
|------|------|------|------|

# At the Barre

## Side knee lifts

**Setup**   Face the barre, one leg bent, knees in line with each other
**Exhale**  Lift knee to side, keep knees in line and do not lift your hip
**Inhale**  Knee back to centre
            Repeat 5 x

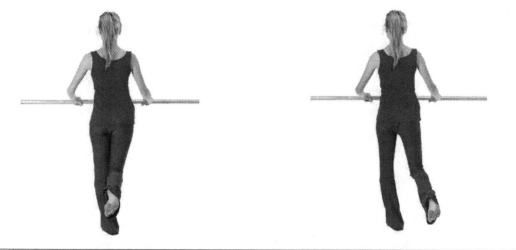

| Do's | Narrow waist throughout exercise<br>Keep hips facing forward | Don'ts | Lift your hips<br>Sink into supporting leg |
|------|-------------------------------------------------------------|--------|---------------------------------------------|

## Back leg extensions

**Setup**   Face the barre, one leg bent, knees in line with each other
**Exhale**  Stretch leg to the back
**Inhale**  Bend leg
            Repeat 5 x

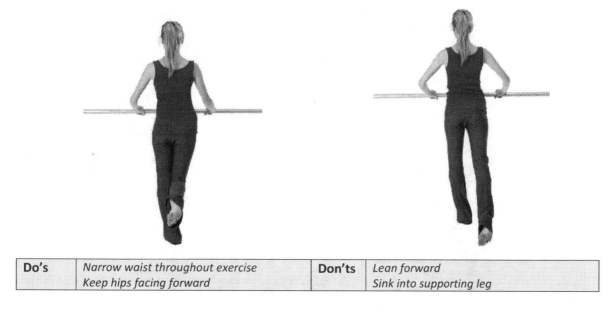

| Do's | Narrow waist throughout exercise<br>Keep hips facing forward | Don'ts | Lean forward<br>Sink into supporting leg |
|------|-------------------------------------------------------------|--------|-------------------------------------------|

## Front knee lift

**Setup**     Face the barre, one leg bent
**Exhale**    Lift knee at front to hip height
**Inhale**     Lower leg
            Repeat 5 x

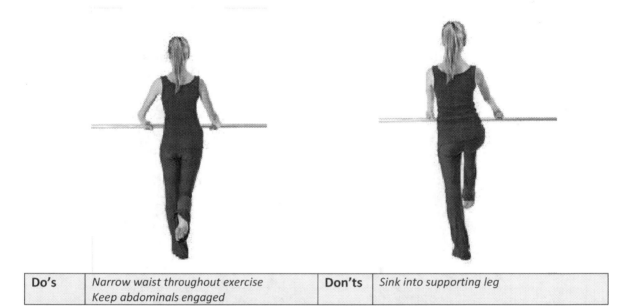

| Do's | Narrow waist throughout exercise<br>Keep abdominals engaged | Don'ts | Sink into supporting leg |
| --- | --- | --- | --- |

## Knee lift to side

**Setup**     Face the barre, one leg bent to front
**Exhale**    Open knee to side
**Inhale**     Back to centre
            Repeat 5 x

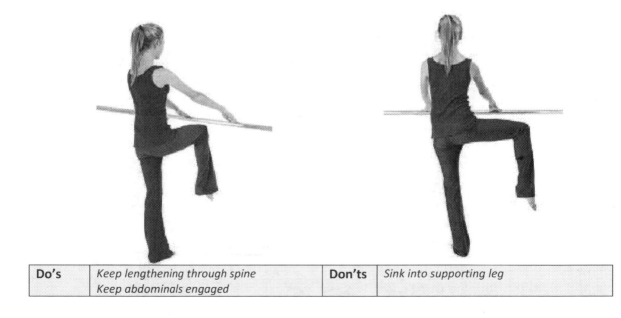

| Do's | Keep lengthening through spine<br>Keep abdominals engaged | Don'ts | Sink into supporting leg |
| --- | --- | --- | --- |

# *Abdominals*

## The 'C' curve

*Before starting the abdominal exercises, let's find the 'C' curve. Sit on the floor with your legs bent, back straight and your feet flat on the floor. Inhale and as you exhale, round your back, keep your shoulders relaxed, pull your abdominals against your spine and feel how you suck in and strengthen your abdominals. Your back is in a long C shape and your spine is lengthened. Inhale and sit up straight.*

*Do not bulge your abdominal muscles. If you bulge your abdominals you will get stronger muscles but your stomach will not flatten.*

## Half roll down

**Setup**   Sitting, legs bent, arms at shoulder level
**Exhale**  Roll back, slide hands on floor in line with hips
**Inhale**  Sit up, arms stretched forward at shoulder level
            Repeat 5 x

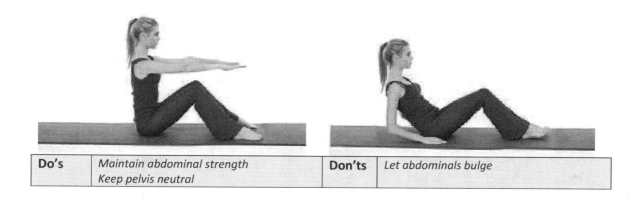

| **Do's** | *Maintain abdominal strength* *Keep pelvis neutral* | **Don'ts** | *Let abdominals bulge* |
|----------|---------------------------------------------------|------------|-----------------------|

## Half roll down with hands on floor

**Setup**   Sitting, legs bent, hands on floor in line with hips
**Exhale**  Roll back, hands stay on floor in line with hips
**Inhale**  Sit up, hands stay on floor
            Repeat 5 x

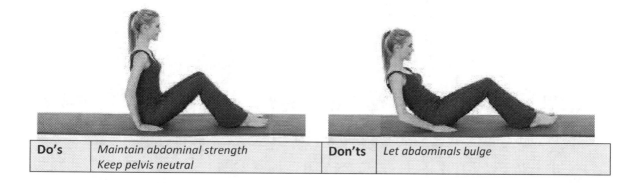

| **Do's** | *Maintain abdominal strength* *Keep pelvis neutral* | **Don'ts** | *Let abdominals bulge* |
|----------|---------------------------------------------------|------------|-----------------------|

## Half roll down with oblique

**Setup**      Sitting, legs bent, arms at shoulder level
**Exhale**     Lean back and place your left then your right elbow on the floor
**Inhale**     Stretch your left then your right arm, stay in 45 degree angle
                  Repeat 5 x left then 5 x right arm

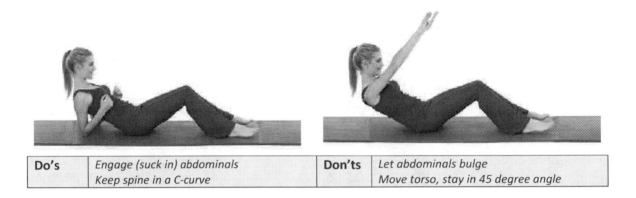

| **Do's** | Engage (suck in) abdominals <br> Keep spine in a C-curve | **Don'ts** | Let abdominals bulge <br> Move torso, stay in 45 degree angle |
|---|---|---|---|

## Teaser preparation

**Setup**      Lying supine, legs 90 degrees, arms stretched overhead, holding hands
**Exhale**     Lift shoulders, drop legs 45 degrees, lift arms overhead, hands touch knees
**Inhale**     Lie down, arms overhead, legs 90 degrees
                  Repeat 10 x

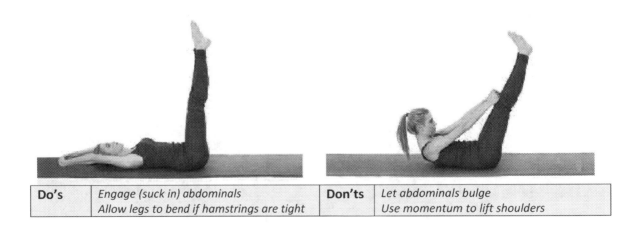

| **Do's** | Engage (suck in) abdominals <br> Allow legs to bend if hamstrings are tight | **Don'ts** | Let abdominals bulge <br> Use momentum to lift shoulders |
|---|---|---|---|

## Shoulder lift with leg extensions

**Setup**    Lying supine, legs in tabletop position, interlace fingers to support neck
**Exhale**    Lift shoulders off floor and push legs out to 45 degrees
**Inhale**    Roll down, legs back to table top position
         Repeat 10 x

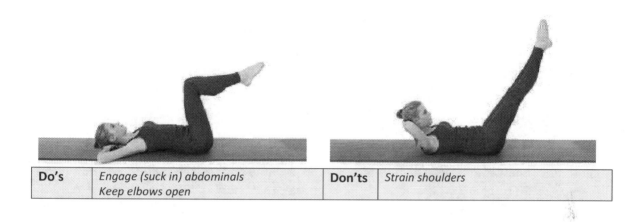

| Do's | Engage (suck in) abdominals<br>Keep elbows open | Don'ts | Strain shoulders |
|---|---|---|---|

## Sitting hundred

**Setup**    Sitting, legs bent, arms in line with shoulders
**Inhale**    Lift legs in tabletop position
         Pump arms up and down in small movements
**Exhale**    Five pumps
**Inhale**    Five pumps
         Repeat 10 x

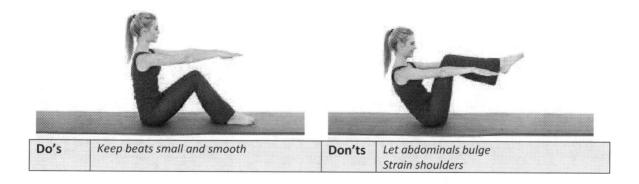

| Do's | Keep beats small and smooth | Don'ts | Let abdominals bulge<br>Strain shoulders |
|---|---|---|---|

# *Side Exercises*

## *Side lift with bent legs*

**Setup**       Lying on side, legs bent, heels in line with buttocks, top arm resting on hip
**Exhale**      Lift body into a straight line
**Inhale**      Down to starting position
               Repeat 5 x

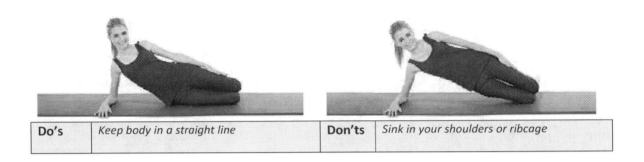

| Do's | Keep body in a straight line | Don'ts | Sink in your shoulders or ribcage |
|------|------------------------------|--------|-----------------------------------|

## *Side lift with leg lift*

**Setup**       Lying on side, bottom leg bent, top leg straight on floor, top arm resting on hip
**Exhale**      Lift body into straight line, lift leg up to hip height, stretch arm
**Inhale**      Down to starting position
               Repeat 5 x

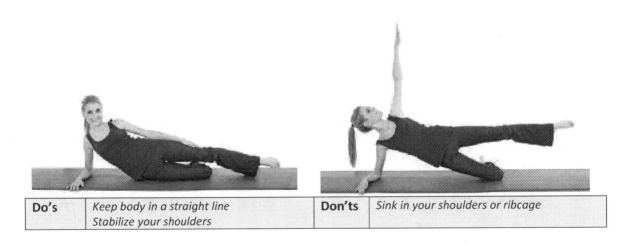

| Do's | Keep body in a straight line<br>Stabilize your shoulders | Don'ts | Sink in your shoulders or ribcage |
|------|----------------------------------------------------------|--------|-----------------------------------|

# Strengthening Exercises

## Side lift with side bend

**Setup**     Sitting, with bottom  leg bent, top leg straight on floor with hand resting on thigh
**Inhale**    Lift hips off floor and stretch arm upwards
**Exhale**    Lift leg hip height and stretch arm into side bend
**Inhale**    Sit down on floor, top leg straight
                   Repeat  5 x

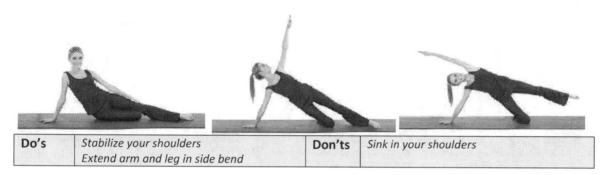

| Do's | Stabilize your shoulders<br>*Extend arm and leg in side bend* | Don'ts | *Sink in your shoulders* |
|------|--------------------------------------------------------------|--------|--------------------------|

## Single leg lift

**Setup**     Sitting, legs bent, feet hip width apart, arms at back fingers facing forward
**Inhale**    Lift hips off floor in tabletop position
**Exhale**    Lift left foot off floor
**Inhale**    Place left foot down on floor
**Exhale**    Lift right foot off floor
                   Repeat 10 x alternating feet

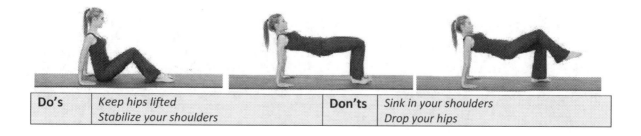

| Do's | Keep hips lifted<br>*Stabilize your shoulders* | Don'ts | *Sink in your shoulders*<br>*Drop your hips* |
|------|-----------------------------------------------|--------|----------------------------------------------|

## Full body stretch

**Setup**    Sitting with both legs to side, hands on floor
**Exhale**   Push up and press heels into the floor
**Inhale**   Sit down on floor and face opposite side
             Repeat 10 x alternating sides

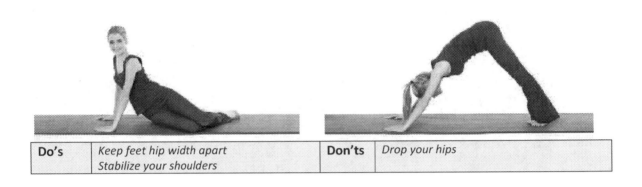

| Do's | Keep feet hip width apart<br>Stabilize your shoulders | Don'ts | Drop your hips |
| --- | --- | --- | --- |

## Front support with knee bends

**Setup**    Kneeling with hands on floor in line with shoulders
**Inhale**   Stretch both legs, body in a straight line
**Exhale**   Bend knees towards floor, do not touch floor
**Inhale**   Stretch legs, keeping body straight
             Repeat 10 x

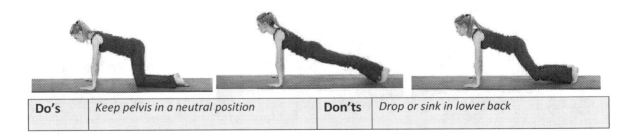

| Do's | Keep pelvis in a neutral position | Don'ts | Drop or sink in lower back |
| --- | --- | --- | --- |

# Spinal Rolls

## Short spine

| | |
|---|---|
| **Setup** | Lying supine, legs at 45 degrees, palms on floor |
| **Exhale** | Roll over and extend toes towards the floor |
| **Inhale** | Bend legs and place knees on floor on either side of your head |
| **Exhale** | Stretch legs out |
| **Inhale** | Bend legs |
| **Exhale** | Stretch legs out |
| **Inhale** | Lift legs parallel and roll back to 45 degrees |
| | Repeat 5 x |

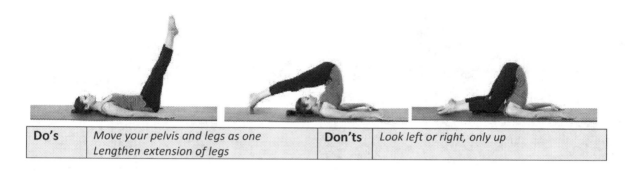

| Do's | Move your pelvis and legs as one<br>Lengthen extension of legs | Don'ts | Look left or right, only up |
|---|---|---|---|

## Roll over with leg extensions

| | |
|---|---|
| **Setup** | Lying supine, holding ankles |
| **Exhale** | Slowly pull your legs over your body  toes on floor |
| **Inhale** | Don't move |
| **Exhale** | Extend your arms, take your toes and extend your legs |
| **Inhale** | Roll back to starting position |
| | Repeat 5 x |

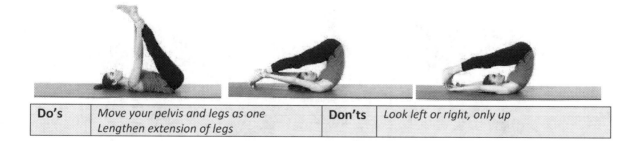

| Do's | Move your pelvis and legs as one<br>Lengthen extension of legs | Don'ts | Look left or right, only up |
|---|---|---|---|

# Spinal Twist

## Spinal twist with leg extension

| | |
|---|---|
| **Setup** | Lying supine, knees bent, arms spread in T-position, palms on floor |
| **Exhale** | Roll over to left side until knees touch floor looking at right hand |
| | Slowly stretch right leg out at 90 degree angle |
| **Inhale** | Bend right leg and roll back to start position |
| | Repeat 10 x alternating sides |

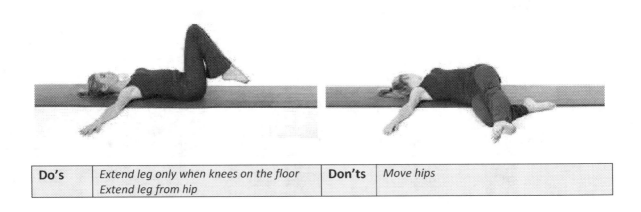

| **Do's** | Extend leg only when knees on the floor | **Don'ts** | Move hips |
|---|---|---|---|
| | Extend leg from hip | | |

## Spinal twist with bent knees

| | |
|---|---|
| **Setup** | Lying supine, knees bent, arms spread in T-position, palms on floor |
| **Exhale** | Roll over to left side until knees touch floor |
| **Inhale** | Roll back to start position |
| **Exhale** | Roll over to right side until knees touch floor |
| **Inhale** | Roll back to start position |
| | Repeat 10 x |

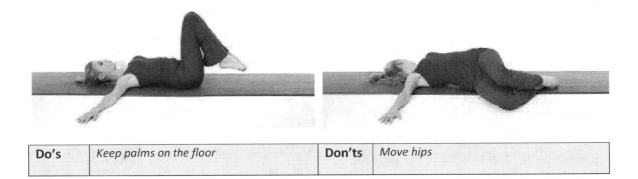

| **Do's** | Keep palms on the floor | **Don'ts** | Move hips |
|---|---|---|---|

# Back Exercises

*When doing back exercises imagine a mirror on the floor and lie with your forehead on the mirror.  As you lift your upper body always look at yourself in the mirror, keep your head in line with your body and let your neck extend from your spine.*

## Push ups

**Setup**  Lying prone, hands in line with shoulders, legs bent, knees apart, soles together
**Exhale**  Extend arms and lift upper body
**Inhale**  Bend arms and lower body
Repeat 5 x

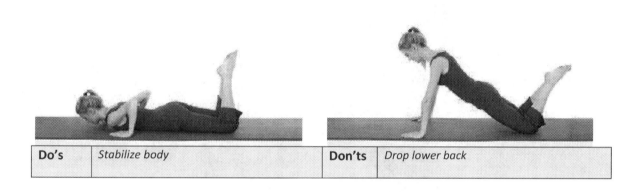

| **Do's** | Stabilize body | **Don'ts** | Drop lower back |
|---|---|---|---|

## Push up with leg extension

**Setup**  Lying prone, hands in line with shoulders
**Exhale**  Push back onto one knee, stretch arms and extend leg
**Inhale**  Return back to start position
Repeat 10 x alternating legs

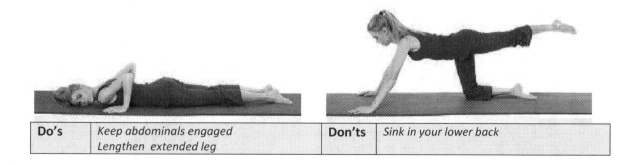

| **Do's** | Keep abdominals engaged<br>Lengthen  extended leg | **Don'ts** | Sink in your lower back |
|---|---|---|---|

# Big Ball

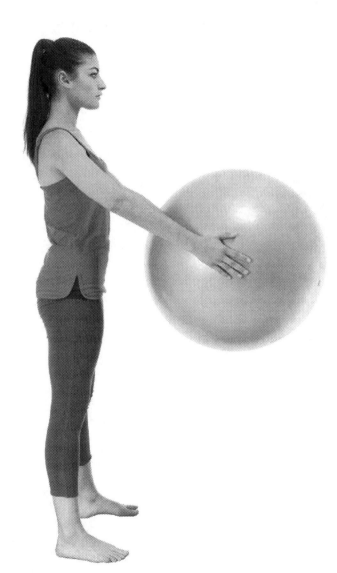

*Perform your work with
minimum effort
and maximum pleasure*

*Joseph Pilates*

## Why exercise with a ball?  It . . .

✓ Challenges your muscles due to the instability of the ball

✓ Strengthens your body as a whole

✓ Improves core muscles

✓ Improves posture

✓ Improves balance

✓ Improves coordination

✓ Improves flexibility

✓ Improves joint mobility

✓ Increases the intensity of the exercises

*And it improves your sense of having fun!!!*

## Choosing the correct ball size

Sit on the ball with your feet flat on the floor.  Your knees should bend at a 90 degree angle or slightly less.  A firmly inflated ball will be more challenging to use than a slightly under inflated ball.  When trying out new exercises, it will be safer to try them with a slightly under inflated ball.

# Warming Up

## Opening the chest

| | |
|---|---|
| **Setup** | Sitting upright on the ball, hands at back on ball, fingers facing down |
| **Exhale** | Push on the ball and stretch out your spine, looking up to the ceiling |
| **Inhale** | Relax |
| | Repeat 5 x |

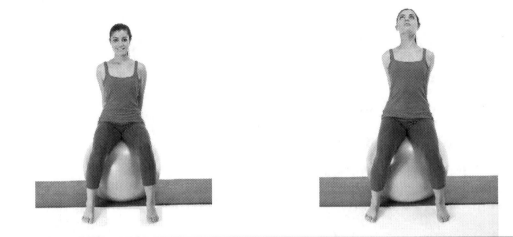

| Do's | Keep shoulders down | Don'ts | Arch into your spine |
|---|---|---|---|
| | *Lengthen torso from waist* | | *Throw head backwards* |

## Arm reach

| | |
|---|---|
| **Setup** | Sitting on ball, fingers interlaced, arms at shoulder level |
| **Exhale** | Round back and extend arms forward |
| **Inhale** | Release arms |
| **Exhale** | Take arms to back, hands interlaced and lift up, open your chest |
| | Repeat 5 x |

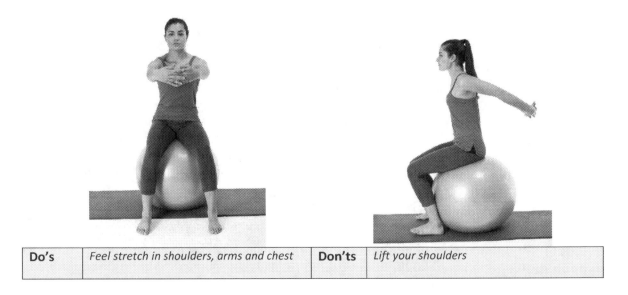

| Do's | Feel stretch in shoulders, arms and chest | Don'ts | Lift your shoulders |
|---|---|---|---|

# *Strengthening Exercises*

## *Forward lunge*

**Setup**    Standing with feet together, holding ball in front
**Exhale**   Step forward into lunge, stretch arms up to the ceiling, bend both legs
**Inhale**   Step backward legs together
              Repeat 10 x alternating legs
              *Do above exercise lunging backwards*

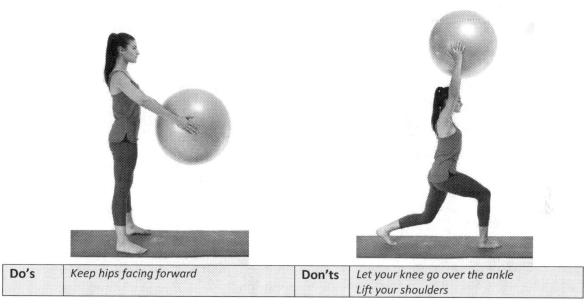

| Do's | Keep hips facing forward | Don'ts | Let your knee go over the ankle |
|------|--------------------------|--------|---------------------------------|
|      |                          |        | Lift your shoulders             |

## *Back support with leg extension*

**Setup**    Lie on ball with head secure on ball, hands on thighs
**Exhale**   Push back and stretch your leg
**Inhale**   Place foot on floor
              Repeat 10 x alternating legs

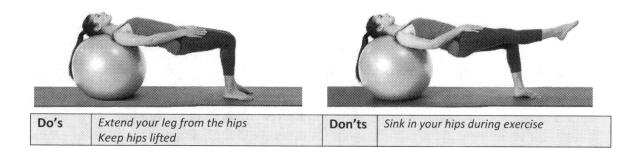

| Do's | Extend your leg from the hips | Don'ts | Sink in your hips during exercise |
|------|-------------------------------|--------|-----------------------------------|
|      | Keep hips lifted              |        |                                   |

# *At the wall*

## *Back extensions*

**Setup**    Lying supine with hips on the ball, feet against the wall
**Inhale**   Hang over ball, arms relaxed
**Exhale**   Lift body up, arms extended to the back
**Inhale**   Hang over the ball
         Repeat 10 x

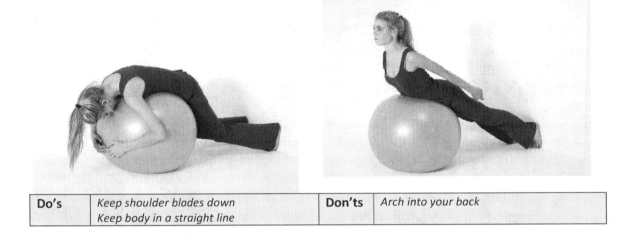

| Do's | Keep shoulder blades down<br>Keep body in a straight line | Don'ts | Arch into your back |
|---|---|---|---|

## *Walking plank*

**Setup**    Place the ball against the wall, hands on the ball, body in a straight line
**Exhale**   Bend knee in to touch ball
**Inhale**   Stretch leg back into plank position
         Repeat 10 x alternating legs

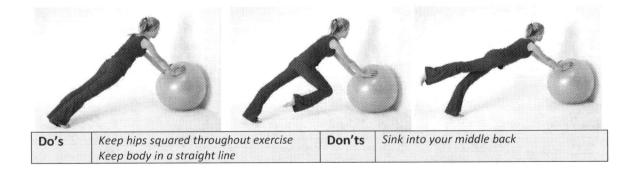

| Do's | Keep hips squared throughout exercise<br>Keep body in a straight line | Don'ts | Sink into your middle back |
|---|---|---|---|

# Abdominals

## Abdominals with double leg stretch

**Setup**   Lying supine, heels on ball, interlace fingers to support your head
**Inhale**   Push legs forward, do not stretch
**Exhale**   Pull back and lift shoulders – small movements, keep your elbows open
              Repeat 10 x

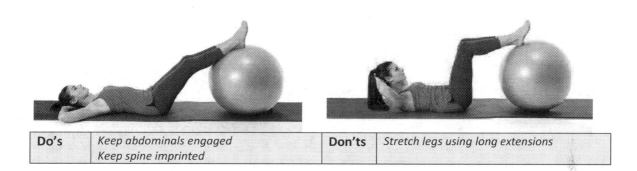

| **Do's** | Keep abdominals engaged<br>Keep spine imprinted | **Don'ts** | Stretch legs using long extensions |
|---|---|---|---|

## Pelvic curl with leg circles

**Setup**   Lying supine, legs bent, feet on ball, palms on floor
**Inhale**   Inhale to prepare and lift hips off floor
**Exhale**   Circle ball clockwise
**Inhale**   Hold position
              Repeat 10 x alternating circles

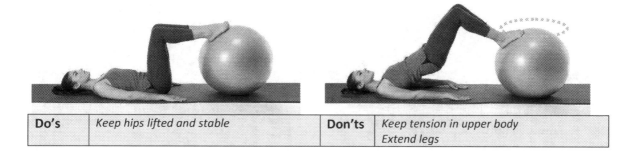

| **Do's** | Keep hips lifted and stable | **Don'ts** | Keep tension in upper body<br>Extend legs |
|---|---|---|---|

## Side to side roll

| | |
|---|---|
| **Setup** | Lying supine, ball close to your body, drape legs over ball, arms to sides |
| **Exhale** | Roll ball over to left side |
| **Inhale** | Back to centre |
| **Exhale** | Roll over to right side |
| | Repeat 10 x alternating sides |

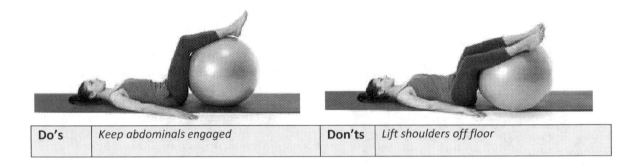

| Do's | Keep abdominals engaged | Don'ts | Lift shoulders off floor |
|---|---|---|---|

## Pelvic curl with arm circles

| | |
|---|---|
| **Setup** | Lying supine, feet on ball, palms on floor |
| **Exhale** | Roll spine off floor, circle arms overhead to back |
| **Inhale** | Roll spine down to floor, arms to front, palms on floor |
| | Repeat 10 x |

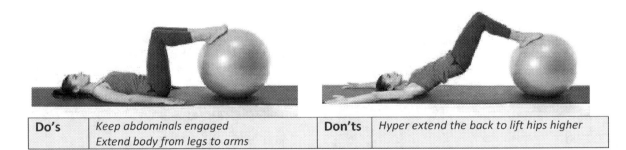

| Do's | Keep abdominals engaged<br>Extend body from legs to arms | Don'ts | Hyper extend the back to lift hips higher |
|---|---|---|---|

## Chest lift

| | |
|---|---|
| **Setup** | Lying supine, ball resting on your chest |
| **Exhale** | Lift shoulders and push ball upwards, feet flexed |
| **Inhale** | Lie down |
| | Repeat 5 x, pulse 10 x |

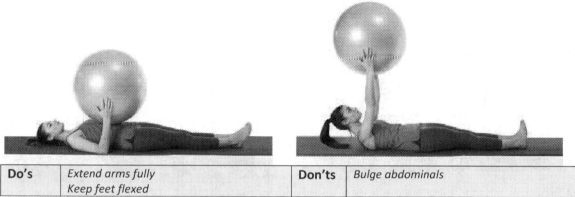

| **Do's** | *Extend arms fully*<br>*Keep feet flexed* | **Don'ts** | *Bulge abdominals* |
|---|---|---|---|

## Abdominal crunch

| | |
|---|---|
| **Setup** | Kneeling, elbows resting on ball, fingers interlaced |
| **Exhale** | Lift knees off floor, press elbows into ball |
| **Inhale** | Lower knees to floor |
| | Repeat 10 x |

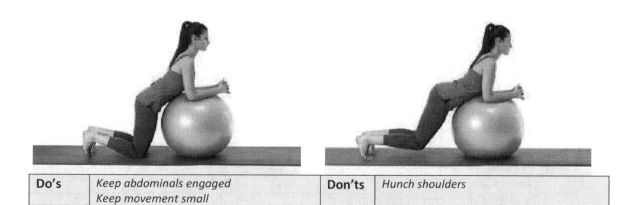

| **Do's** | *Keep abdominals engaged*<br>*Keep movement small* | **Don'ts** | *Hunch shoulders* |
|---|---|---|---|

## Teaser prep

| | |
|---|---|
| **Setup** | Sitting, legs bent, ball resting on shins |
| **Exhale** | Lift legs to tabletop and stretch arms upwards holding the ball |
| **Inhale** | Return to start position |
| | Repeat 10 x |

| Do's | Keep abdominals engaged<br>Articulate up and down through the spine | Don'ts | Let abdominals bulge<br>Lift your shoulders |
|---|---|---|---|

## Teaser with oblique

| | |
|---|---|
| **Setup** | Sitting, legs bent, arms stretched upwards holding the ball |
| **Exhale** | Lift legs to V position, ball to left side |
| **Inhale** | Bend legs and stretch arms |
| **Exhale** | Lift legs to V position, ball to right side |
| | Repeat 10 x alternating sides |

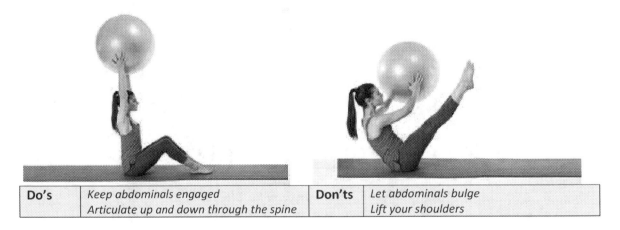

| Do's | Keep abdominals engaged<br>Articulate up and down through the spine | Don'ts | Let abdominals bulge<br>Lift your shoulders |
|---|---|---|---|

# *Sides and Butt*

## *Side leg lifts with forward roll*

**Setup**   Lying on side, ball between legs
**Inhale**  Inhale to prepare and lift legs off floor
**Exhale**  Roll ball forward, keep legs lifted
**Inhale**  Roll ball backwards
         Repeat 10 x

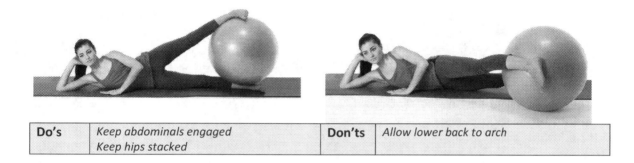

| Do's | Keep abdominals engaged<br>Keep hips stacked | Don'ts | *Allow lower back to arch* |
|------|-----------------------------------------------|--------|----------------------------|

## *Kneeling knee bend*

**Setup**   Kneeling on side of ball, leaning over ball, leg stretched to side
**Exhale**  Bend knee in to touch ball, keeping leg parallel to floor
**Inhale**  Stretch leg out touching the floor
         Repeat 10 x

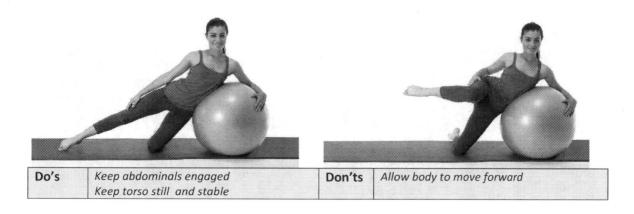

| Do's | Keep abdominals engaged<br>Keep torso still and stable | Don'ts | *Allow body to move forward* |
|------|---------------------------------------------------------|--------|------------------------------|

## Kneeling with leg lift

**Setup**    Kneeling on side of ball, leaning over ball, leg stretched to side
**Exhale**   Lift leg slightly higher than hip height
**Inhale**   Lower leg down to floor
             Repeat 10 x

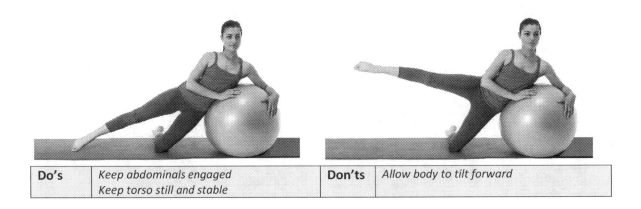

| Do's | Keep abdominals engaged<br>Keep torso still and stable | Don'ts | Allow body to tilt forward |
|------|-------------------------------------------------------|--------|----------------------------|

## Kneeling with side kicks

**Setup**    Kneeling on side of ball, leaning over ball, leg lifted to hip height
**Exhale**   Swing leg forward with foot flexed
**Inhale**   Swing leg backward with toes pointed
             Repeat 10 x

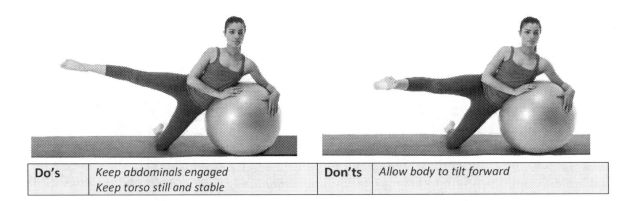

| Do's | Keep abdominals engaged<br>Keep torso still and stable | Don'ts | Allow body to tilt forward |
|------|-------------------------------------------------------|--------|----------------------------|

## Hip lift on ball

**Setup**   Lying with lower back and head supported on ball, legs bent, hands resting on thighs
**Exhale**  Lift hips to tabletop
**Inhale**  Lower hips
            Repeat 10 x

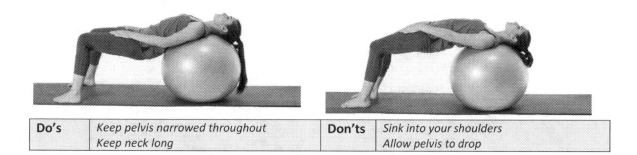

| **Do's** | Keep pelvis narrowed throughout<br>Keep neck long | **Don'ts** | Sink into your shoulders<br>Allow pelvis to drop |
|---|---|---|---|

## Leg squeezes

**Setup**   Lying with lower back and head supported on ball, legs bent, feet wide apart, hands resting on thighs
**Exhale**  Knees together
**Inhale**  Knees open
            Repeat 10 x

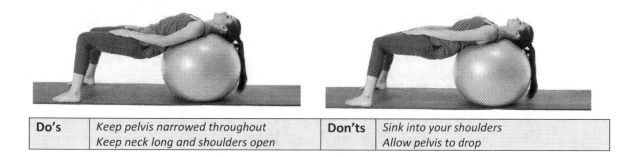

| **Do's** | Keep pelvis narrowed throughout<br>Keep neck long and shoulders open | **Don'ts** | Sink into your shoulders<br>Allow pelvis to drop |
|---|---|---|---|

# *Spinal Rolls*

## *Boomerang*

| | |
|---|---|
| **Setup** | Sitting, legs bent, holding ball in hands |
| **Exhale** | Roll backwards and place feet on ball, palms on floor |
| **Inhale** | Take ball and roll back to start position |
| | Repeat 5 x |

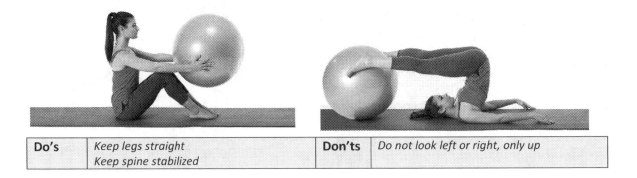

| Do's | Keep legs straight<br>Keep spine stabilized | Don'ts | *Do not look left or right, only up* |
|---|---|---|---|

## *Roll over with leg extension*

| | |
|---|---|
| **Setup** | Roll backwards and place feet on ball, palms on floor |
| **Exhale** | Bend your legs, roll ball towards you |
| **Inhale** | Straighten your legs, roll ball away from you |
| | Repeat 10 x |

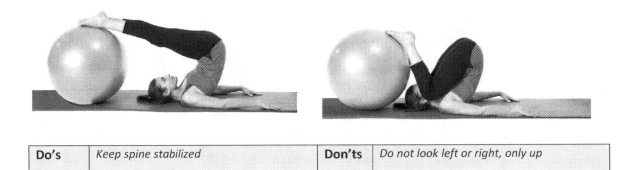

| Do's | Keep spine stabilized | Don'ts | *Do not look left or right, only up* |
|---|---|---|---|

## Roll over

**Setup**   Lying supine, legs at 45 degrees, ball between feet, palms on floor
**Exhale**  Roll legs over head and place ball on floor
**Inhale**  Hold position
**Exhale**  Slowly roll legs back to start position
            Repeat 10 x

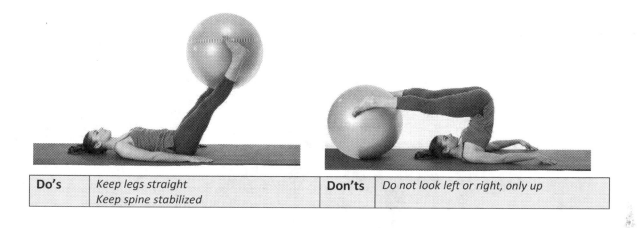

| Do's | Keep legs straight | Don'ts | Do not look left or right, only up |
|------|--------------------|--------|-----------------------------------|
|      | Keep spine stabilized |     |                                   |

## Spinal twist

**Setup**   Lying supine, legs bent, holding ball in both hands
**Exhale**  Roll legs over to left side and arms to right side, look at ball
**Inhale**  Roll back to starting position
            Repeat 10 x alternating sides

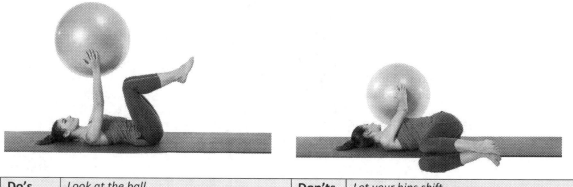

| Do's | Look at the ball | Don'ts | Let your hips shift |
|------|------------------|--------|---------------------|
|      | Knees must touch the floor | | Let your feet touch the floor |

# Small Ball

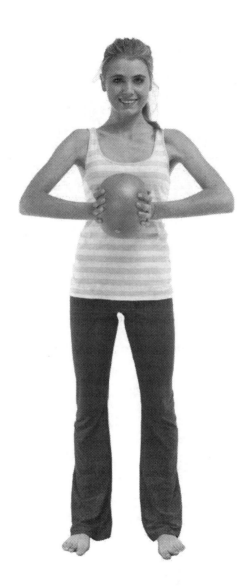

*Physical fitness is the first prerequisite to happiness*

*Joseph Pilates*

## *Why exercise with a small ball?*

For the same reasons we use the big ball.  It . . .

✓ Challenges your muscles due to the instability of the ball

✓ Strengthens your body as a whole

✓ Improves core muscles

✓ Improves posture

✓ Improves balance

✓ Improves coordination

✓ Improves flexibility

✓ Improves joint mobility

✓ Increases the intensity of the exercises

# Warming Up

## Standing roll down

**Setup**    Standing, feet hip width apart, holding ball with both hands
**Exhale**   Roll ball down to the floor and away from your body
**Inhale**    Roll ball up into start position
             Repeat 5 x

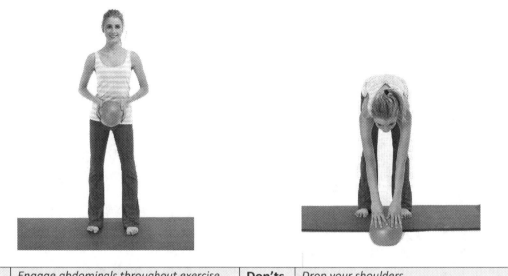

| Do's | Engage abdominals throughout exercise<br>Keep weight even over both feet | Don'ts | Drop your shoulders |
|------|--------------------------------------------------------------------------|--------|---------------------|

## Shoulder stabilisation

**Setup**    Standing, feet hip width apart, holding ball with both hands on chest
**Exhale**   Squeeze ball with both hands
**Inhale**    Relax
             Repeat 10 x

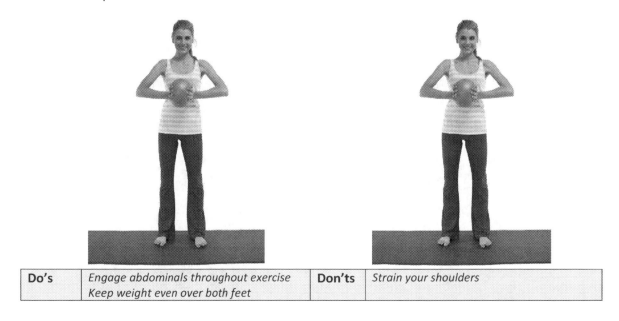

| Do's | Engage abdominals throughout exercise<br>Keep weight even over both feet | Don'ts | Strain your shoulders |
|------|--------------------------------------------------------------------------|--------|-----------------------|

# *Abdominals*

## *Passing the ball prep*

**Setup**     Sitting, legs bent, holding ball in right hand
**Exhale**   Lift legs into tabletop, pass ball under knees to left hand
**Inhale**   Place feet on floor
              Repeat 10 x passing ball from hand to hand

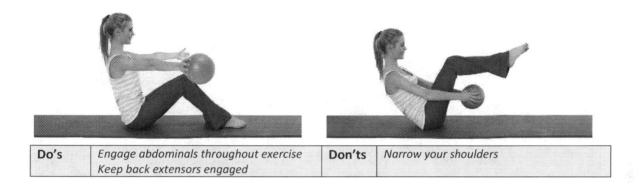

| Do's | Engage abdominals throughout exercise<br>Keep back extensors engaged | Don'ts | Narrow your shoulders |
|------|------|------|------|

## *Passing the ball*

**Setup**     Sitting, legs bent, holding ball in right hand
**Exhale**   Lift legs into V position, pass ball under knees to left hand
**Inhale**   Place feet on floor
              Repeat 10 x passing ball from hand to hand

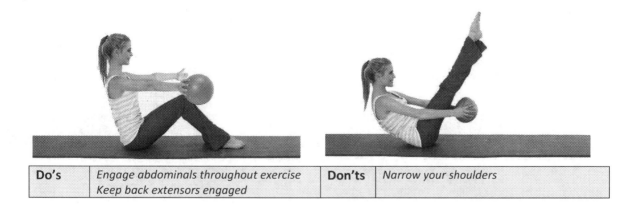

| Do's | Engage abdominals throughout exercise<br>Keep back extensors engaged | Don'ts | Narrow your shoulders |
|------|------|------|------|

## Half roll down

**Setup**     Sitting, legs bent, ball placed at lower back, arms stretched forward
**Exhale**    Roll back, open arms to sides
**Inhale**    Sit up, do not lose contact with ball
            Repeat 5 x

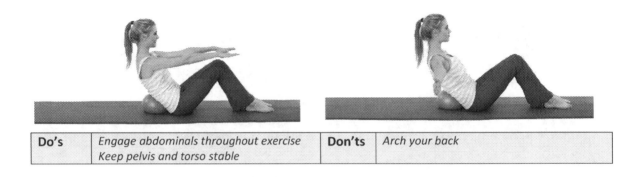

| Do's | Engage abdominals throughout exercise Keep pelvis and torso stable | Don'ts | Arch your back |
|------|------|------|------|

## Half roll down with arm extensions

**Setup**     Sitting, legs bent, ball placed at lower back, arms stretched forward
**Exhale**    Roll back, stretch arms upwards in line with ears
**Inhale**    Sit up, do not lose contact with ball
            Repeat 5 x

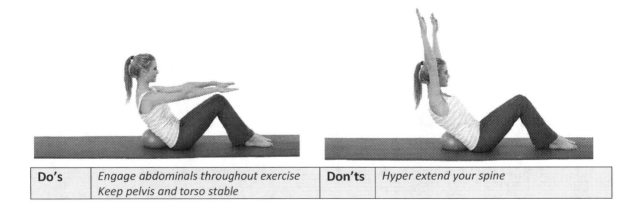

| Do's | Engage abdominals throughout exercise Keep pelvis and torso stable | Don'ts | Hyper extend your spine |
|------|------|------|------|

## Teaser prep

**Setup**   Sitting, legs bent, ball placed at lower back, fingers interlaced supporting neck
**Inhale**   Lean back, bend knee to chest
**Exhale**   Stretch leg to floor
Repeat 10 x alternating sides

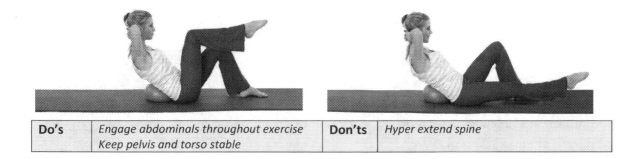

| Do's | Engage abdominals throughout exercise<br>Keep pelvis and torso stable | Don'ts | Hyper extend spine |
| --- | --- | --- | --- |

## Chest lift

**Setup**   Lying, legs bent, ball placed between shoulder blades, fingers interlaced supporting neck
**Exhale**   Lift shoulders, keep elbows open, do not lose contact with ball
**Inhale**   Lie back down on ball
Repeat 10 x

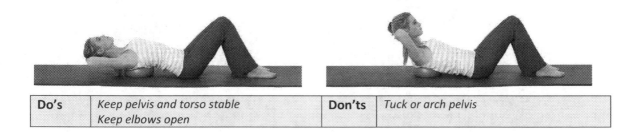

| Do's | Keep pelvis and torso stable<br>Keep elbows open | Don'ts | Tuck or arch pelvis |
| --- | --- | --- | --- |

## Chest lift with arm extensions

**Setup**   Lying, legs bent, ball placed between shoulder blades, hand supporting neck
**Inhale**  Stretch left arm in line with ear, lie back on ball, open chest
**Exhale**  Lift shoulders, touch right knee with left hand, do not lose touch with ball
**Inhale**  Lie back on ball
              Repeat 10 x alternating arms

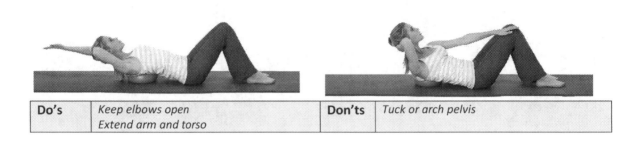

| Do's | Keep elbows open<br>Extend arm and torso | Don'ts | Tuck or arch pelvis |
|------|------------------------------------------|--------|---------------------|

## Leg changes

**Setup**   Lying supine, ball under pelvis, legs in tabletop
**Exhale**  Tap left toe on floor 2 x
**Inhale**  Legs to tabletop
**Exhale**  Tap right toe on floor 2 x
              Repeat 10 x alternating legs

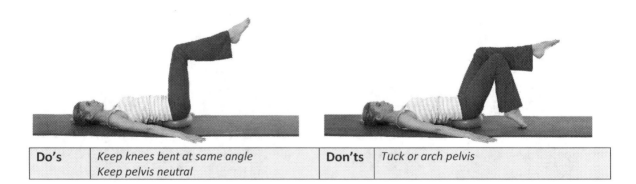

| Do's | Keep knees bent at same angle<br>Keep pelvis neutral | Don'ts | Tuck or arch pelvis |
|------|------------------------------------------------------|--------|---------------------|

## Single leg extensions

**Setup**   Lying supine, legs 90 degrees, ball under pelvis, palms on floor
**Exhale**  Flex feet and take your leg straight down
**Inhale**  Lift leg to 90 degrees
        Repeat 10 x alternating legs

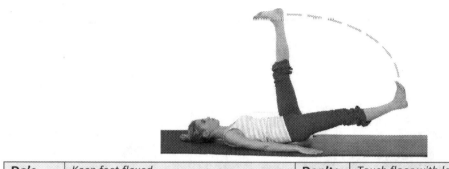

| Do's | Keep feet flexed<br>Keep pelvis neutral | Don'ts | Touch floor with lower leg, keep hip height |
|------|------------------------------------------|--------|----------------------------------------------|

## Roll over prep

**Setup**   Lying supine, legs bent with ball under knees, palms on floor
**Exhale**  Push body up keeping knees bent
**Inhale**  Roll down to start position
        Repeat 10 x

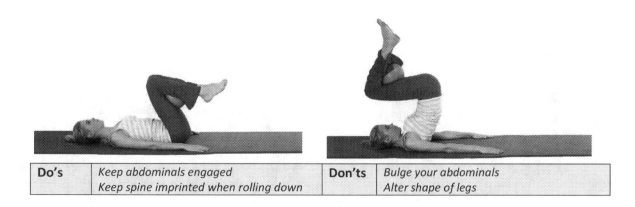

| Do's | Keep abdominals engaged<br>Keep spine imprinted when rolling down | Don'ts | Bulge your abdominals<br>Alter shape of legs |
|------|-------------------------------------------------------------------|--------|-----------------------------------------------|

# Sides and Butt

## Side leg lifts

**Setup**    Lying on side, legs extended with ball between ankles
**Inhale**   Lift legs off floor, squeeze ball between ankles
**Exhale**   Move legs forward with ball between ankles
**Inhale**   Move legs back to start position
             Repeat 10 x

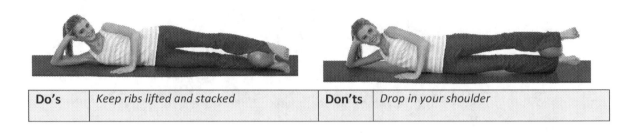

| Do's | Keep ribs lifted and stacked | Don'ts | Drop in your shoulder |
|------|------------------------------|--------|-----------------------|

## Knee to front

**Setup**    Lying on side, leg bent with ball behind knee
**Exhale**   Bring knee forward in line with hips
**Inhale**   Push leg backwards
             Repeat 10 x

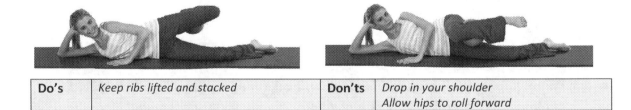

| Do's | Keep ribs lifted and stacked | Don'ts | Drop in your shoulder<br>Allow hips to roll forward |
|------|------------------------------|--------|-----------------------------------------------------|

## Bent knee lift

**Setup**   Kneeling, ball behind knee, hands on floor in line with shoulders
**Inhale**  Bring knee towards chest
**Exhale**  Push leg upwards, keeping knee bent
           Repeat 10 x and pulse 10 x

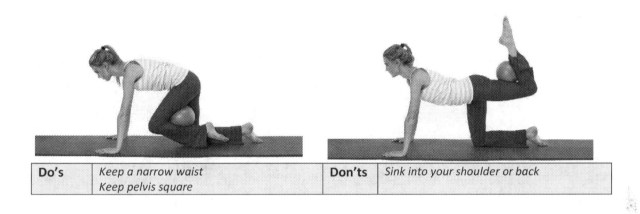

| Do's | Keep a narrow waist<br>Keep pelvis square | Don'ts | Sink into your shoulder or back |
|------|-------------------------------------------|--------|----------------------------------|

## Side knee lift

**Setup**   Kneeling on left knee with hand on floor in line with hip, ball behind right knee
**Inhale**  Lift knee hip height to side
**Exhale**  Bring knee forward in line with hips
**Inhale**  Take knee backwards
           Repeat 10 x

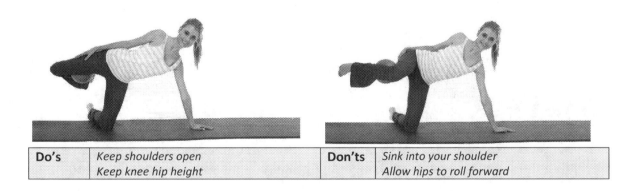

| Do's | Keep shoulders open<br>Keep knee hip height | Don'ts | Sink into your shoulder<br>Allow hips to roll forward |
|------|---------------------------------------------|--------|--------------------------------------------------------|

# Spinal Rolls

## Roll over

| | |
|---|---|
| **Setup** | Sitting, legs stretched forward, ball between ankles |
| **Inhale** | Reach forward |
| **Exhale** | Roll backwards, touch toes on floor |
| **Inhale** | Roll back to start position |
| | Repeat 5 x |

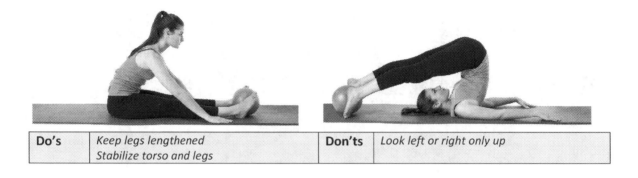

| **Do's** | Keep legs lengthened<br>Stabilize torso and legs | **Don'ts** | Look left or right only up |
|---|---|---|---|

## Spinal twist

| | |
|---|---|
| **Setup** | Lying supine, legs bent, ball between knees, arms open to sides, palms on floor |
| **Exhale** | Roll over to side, touch knee to floor, looking at opposite hand |
| **Inhale** | Roll back to centre |
| | Repeat 10 x alternating sides |

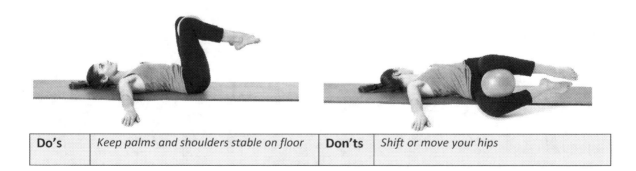

| **Do's** | Keep palms and shoulders stable on floor | **Don'ts** | Shift or move your hips |
|---|---|---|---|

# Back Exercises

## Ball squeeze

**Setup**   Lying prone, chin resting on hands, ball between ankles
**Exhale**  Stretch legs out and squeeze the ball
**Inhale**  Relax
Repeat 5 x

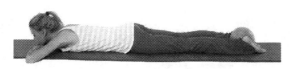

| Do's | *Keep pelvis narrowed to avoid sinking your back* | Don'ts | *Lift legs* |
|------|---------------------------------------------------|--------|-------------|

## Double leg lift

**Setup**   Lying prone, chin resting on hands, legs bent, ball between ankles
**Exhale**  Push legs upwards,  and squeeze the ball
**Inhale**  Relax
Repeat 5 x

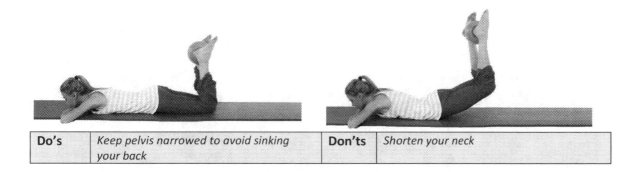

| Do's | *Keep pelvis narrowed to avoid sinking your back* | Don'ts | *Shorten your neck* |
|------|---------------------------------------------------|--------|---------------------|

## Single leg push up

| | |
|---|---|
| **Setup** | Lying prone, chin resting on hands, left leg bent, ball in bent knee |
| **Exhale** | Push leg upwards keeping knee bent |
| **Inhale** | Relax leg onto floor |
| | Repeat 5 x |

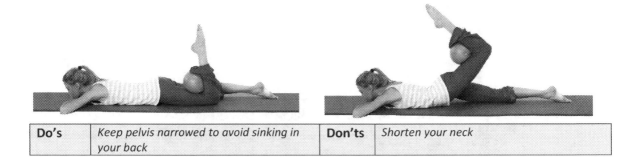

| Do's | Keep pelvis narrowed to avoid sinking in your back | Don'ts | Shorten your neck |
|---|---|---|---|

## Back extension passing the ball

| | |
|---|---|
| **Setup** | Lying prone, arms stretched forward holding ball in left hand |
| **Inhale** | Lift torso, pass ball at back to right hand |
| **Exhale** | Relax to start position |
| **Inhale** | Lift torso and pass ball at back to left hand |
| | Repeat 10 x changing hands |

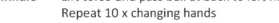

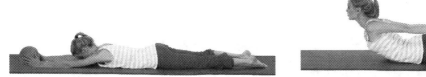
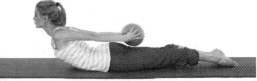

| Do's | Keep arms lengthened<br>Keep abdominals lifted | Don'ts | Shorten your neck<br>Strain neck and shoulders |
|---|---|---|---|

*To achieve the highset accomplishments*

*within the scope of our capabilities in all*

*walks of life, we must constantly strive to*

*acquire strong, healthy bodies and develop*

*our minds to the limits of our ability.*

*Joseph Pilates*

# Pilates Ring

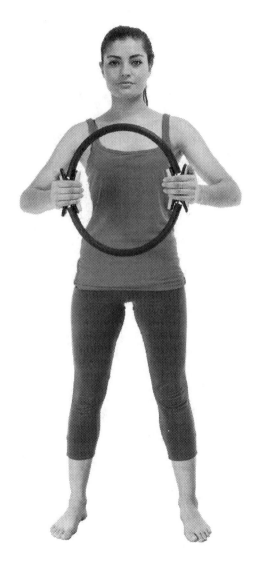

*Patience and persistence are vital qualities
in the ultimate successful accomplishment
of any worthwhile endeavour*

*Joseph Pilates*

## *Why exercise with the Pilates Ring?*

- ✓ It provides resistance

- ✓ Intensifies all of the exercises

- ✓ Improves your coordination

- ✓ Balances your body

- ✓ Improves muscle tone

# *Warming Up*

## *Pectoral stretch*

| | |
|---|---|
| **Setup** | Standing, feet hip width apart, holding ring with both hands |
| **Exhale** | Squeeze ring together |
| **Inhale** | Relax |
| | Repeat 10 x |

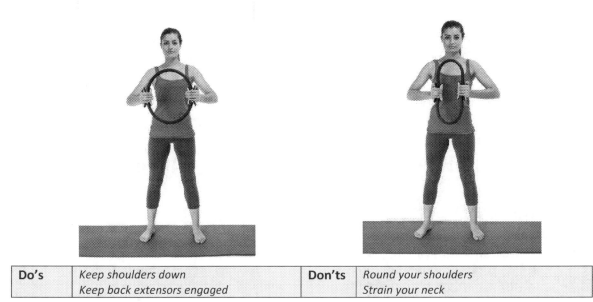

| Do's | Keep shoulders down<br>Keep back extensors engaged | Don'ts | Round your shoulders<br>Strain your neck |
|---|---|---|---|

## *Arms overhead*

| | |
|---|---|
| **Setup** | Standing, feet hip width apart, holding ring with both hands |
| **Exhale** | Lift arms above head, squeeze ring together |
| **Inhale** | Arms down |
| | Repeat 10 x |

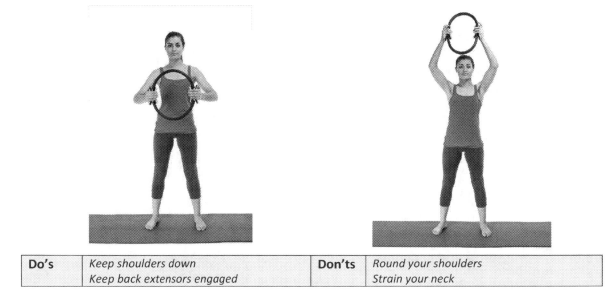

| Do's | Keep shoulders down<br>Keep back extensors engaged | Don'ts | Round your shoulders<br>Strain your neck |
|---|---|---|---|

## *Leg stretch*

| | |
|---|---|
| **Setup** | Standing with one foot in ring, holding ring with both hands |
| **Exhale** | Stretch leg forward keeping body upright |
| **Inhale** | Lower leg |
| | Repeat 5 x |

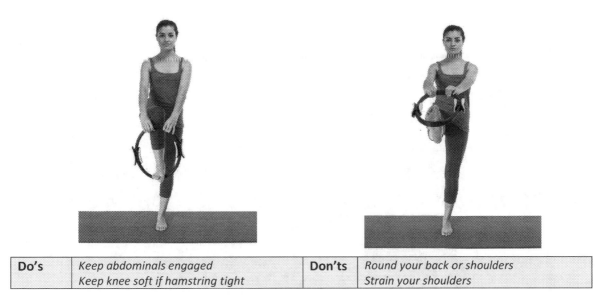

| **Do's** | Keep abdominals engaged<br>Keep knee soft if hamstring tight | **Don'ts** | Round your back or shoulders<br>Strain your shoulders |
|---|---|---|---|

## *Side stretch with leg lift*

| | |
|---|---|
| **Setup** | Standing with feet together, holding ring with both hands |
| **Exhale** | Extend arms to side and lift leg |
| **Inhale** | Feet together, arms down |
| | Repeat 10 x alternating sides |

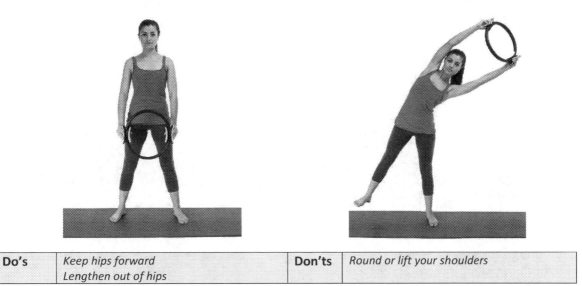

| **Do's** | Keep hips forward<br>Lengthen out of hips | **Don'ts** | Round or lift your shoulders |
|---|---|---|---|

# Abdominals

## Half roll down with leg extension

| | |
|---|---|
| **Setup** | Sitting with one foot in ring, holding ring in both hands |
| **Exhale** | Roll down and stretch leg |
| **Inhale** | Roll up and bend leg |
| | Repeat 5 x |

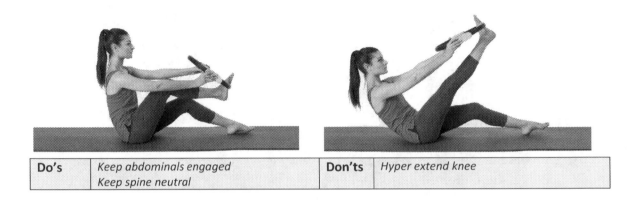

| Do's | Keep abdominals engaged<br>Keep spine neutral | Don'ts | Hyper extend knee |
|---|---|---|---|

## Full roll down

| | |
|---|---|
| **Setup** | Sitting with legs bent, holding ring in both hands |
| **Exhale** | Roll down to floor, stretch arms overhead, place ring on floor |
| **Inhale** | Roll up to start position |
| | Repeat 10 x |

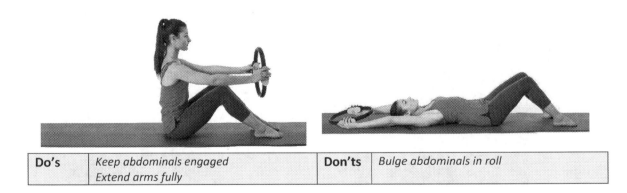

| Do's | Keep abdominals engaged<br>Extend arms fully | Don'ts | Bulge abdominals in roll |
|---|---|---|---|

## Abdominal crunch

| | |
|---|---|
| **Setup** | Lying supine, ring between knees, interlaced fingers supporting head |
| **Exhale** | Lift shoulders, bring knees to chest and squeeze ring |
| **Inhale** | Roll down, place feet on floor |
| | Repeat 10 x |

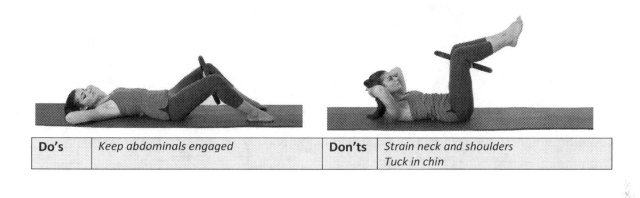

| **Do's** | Keep abdominals engaged | **Don'ts** | Strain neck and shoulders<br>Tuck in chin |
|---|---|---|---|

## Full roll up with straight leg

| | |
|---|---|
| **Setup** | Lying supine, one foot in ring, holding ring with both hands |
| **Exhale** | Roll up to sitting position |
| **Inhale** | Roll down to start position |
| | Repeat 5 x |

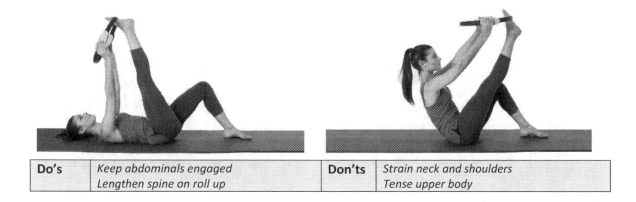

| **Do's** | Keep abdominals engaged<br>Lengthen spine on roll up | **Don'ts** | Strain neck and shoulders<br>Tense upper body |
|---|---|---|---|

## Hundred prep

**Setup**   Lying supine, legs 90 degrees, ring between feet, interlaced fingers supporting head
**Exhale**  Lift shoulders, drop legs to 45 degree angle
**Inhale**  Roll back to start position
            Repeat 10 x

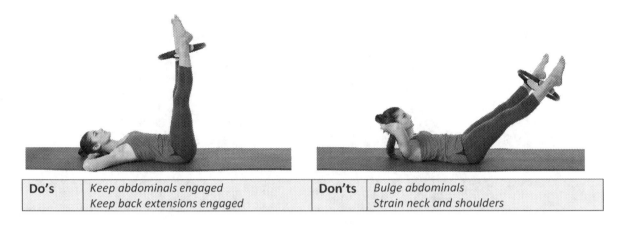

| Do's | Keep abdominals engaged<br>Keep back extensions engaged | Don'ts | Bulge abdominals<br>Strain neck and shoulders |
|------|--------------------------------------------------------|--------|-----------------------------------------------|

## Teaser

**Setup**   Lying supine, ring between feet, palms on floor
**Exhale**  Sit up into V position
**Inhale**  Roll down to start position
            Repeat 5 x

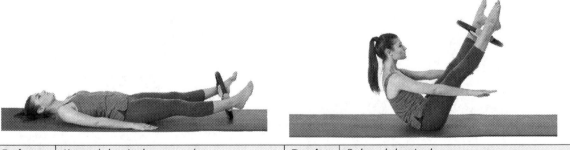

| Do's | Keep abdominals engaged<br>Keep back extensions engaged | Don'ts | Bulge abdominals<br>Strain upper body |
|------|--------------------------------------------------------|--------|---------------------------------------|

# Side Exercises

## Side leg lift

**Setup**   Lying on side,  holding ring between feet,  hand on your hip
**Exhale**   Lift  legs  and stretch your arm upwards
**Inhale**   Relax
          Repeat 10 x

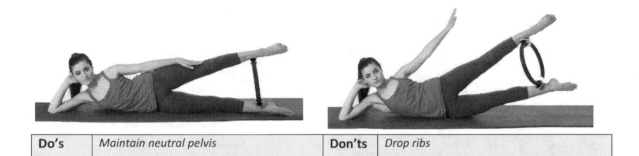

| Do's | Maintain neutral pelvis | Don'ts | Drop ribs |
|------|-------------------------|--------|-----------|

## Tweezer

**Setup**   Lying on side, holding ring between feet, hand on floor
**Exhale**   Slide arm inwards, sit up to a sideways V position
**Inhale**   Slide down to start position
          Repeat 5 x

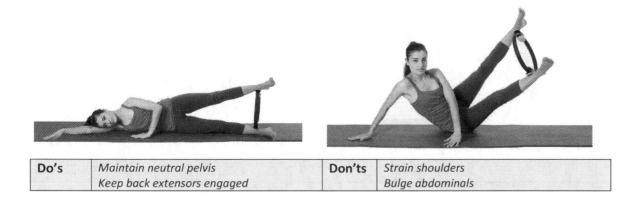

| Do's | Maintain neutral pelvis<br>Keep back extensors engaged | Don'ts | Strain shoulders<br>Bulge abdominals |
|------|-------------------------------------------------------|--------|--------------------------------------|

# Spinal Rolls

## *Roll over*

**Setup**    Lying supine, legs straight, holding ring between feet
**Exhale**   Roll backwards legs parallel to floor
**Inhale**   Roll back to start position
             Repeat 5 x

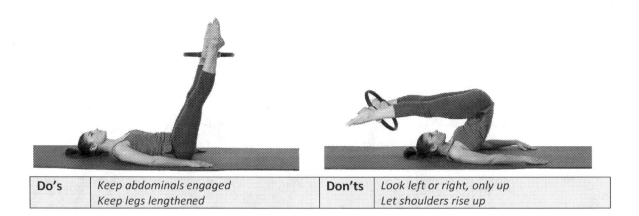

| **Do's** | Keep abdominals engaged | **Don'ts** | Look left or right, only up |
| --- | --- | --- | --- |
|  | Keep legs lengthened |  | Let shoulders rise up |

## *Open leg rocker*

**Setup**    Sitting with legs in a V position, holding ankles, ring between feet
**Exhale**   Roll back, legs parallel to floor
**Inhale**   Roll up to start position
             Repeat 5 x

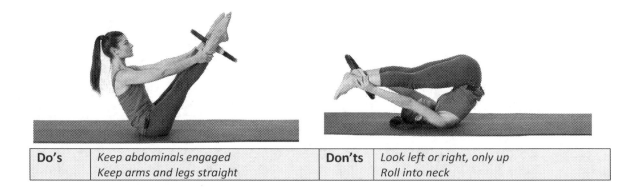

| **Do's** | Keep abdominals engaged | **Don'ts** | Look left or right, only up |
| --- | --- | --- | --- |
|  | Keep arms and legs straight |  | Roll into neck |

# Back Exercises

## Bent leg squeeze

**Setup**  Lying prone, legs bent, holding ring between feet
**Exhale**  Squeeze ring
**Inhale**  Relax
 Repeat 10 x

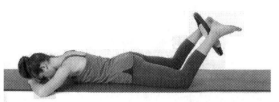

| Do's | Press inwards with both legs<br>*Keep back extensions engaged* | Don'ts | *Sink into lower back* |
|------|----------------------------------------------------------------|--------|------------------------|

## Bent leg lift

**Setup**  Lying prone, legs bent, holding ring between feet
**Exhale**  Push legs up
**Inhale**  Relax
 Repeat 10 x

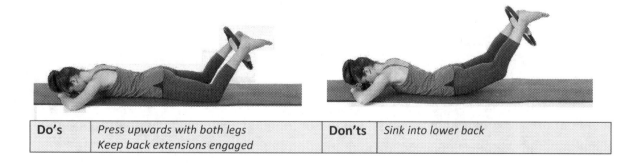

| Do's | Press upwards with both legs<br>*Keep back extensions engaged* | Don'ts | *Sink into lower back* |
|------|----------------------------------------------------------------|--------|------------------------|

# Thera Band

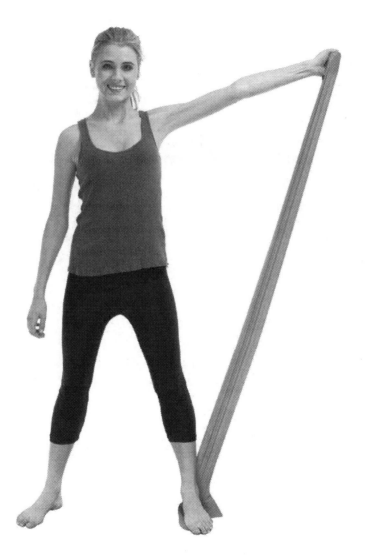

*True flexibility can be achieved
only when all muscles are
uniformly developed*

*Joseph Pilates*

## Why exercise with the Thera Band?

What does your body need, weights or your own body's resistance?
The Thera Band will give you all the resistance your body needs and it will give you …

- ✓ Strength

- ✓ Flexibility

- ✓ Mobility

- ✓ Endurance

- ✓ Enhanced muscle tone

- ✓ Improved bone protection and reduced risk of osteoporosis

- ✓ Prevention of muscle and joint loss caused by ageing

   *The Thera band makes you do MORE!!!*

   **Have fun!!!**

# *Warming Up*

## *Open arm stretch*

| | |
|---|---|
| **Setup** | Standing, feet hip width apart, holding band shoulder height with both hands |
| **Exhale** | Open band |
| **Inhale** | Relax band |
| | Repeat 10 x |

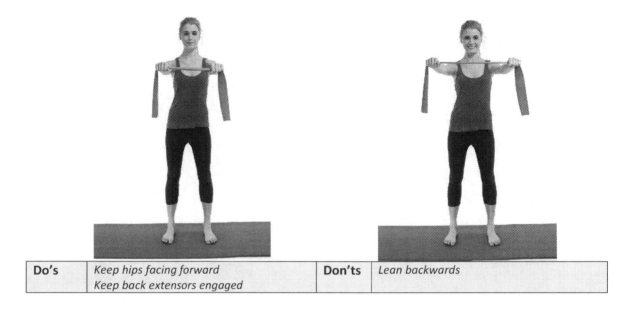

| Do's | *Keep hips facing forward* | Don'ts | *Lean backwards* |
|---|---|---|---|
| | *Keep back extensors engaged* | | |

## *Overhead reach*

| | |
|---|---|
| **Setup** | Standing, feet hip width apart, holding band shoulder height with both hands |
| **Exhale** | Raise arms upwards, stretch band with both hands |
| **Inhale** | Release arms to start position |
| | Repeat 10 x |

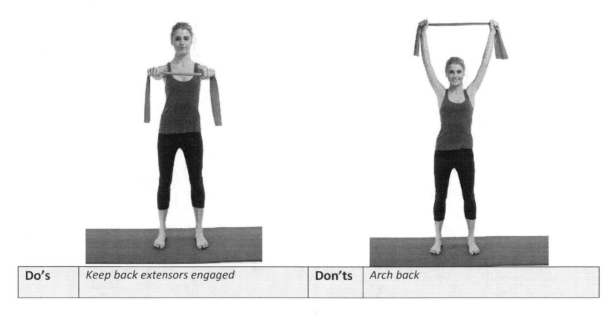

| Do's | *Keep back extensors engaged* | Don'ts | *Arch back* |
|---|---|---|---|

## Chest expansion

| | |
|---|---|
| **Setup** | Standing, feet hip width apart, holding band at back, arms relaxed |
| **Exhale** | Lift arms and open band |
| **Inhale** | Relax |
| | Repeat 10 x |

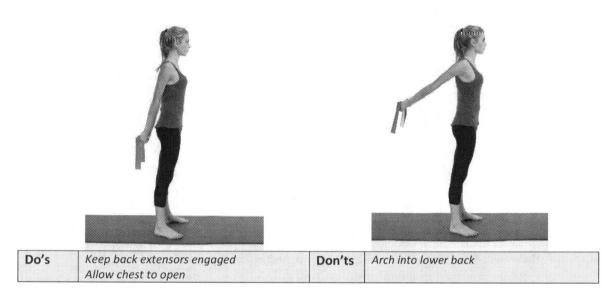

| Do's | Keep back extensors engaged<br>Allow chest to open | Don'ts | Arch into lower back |
|---|---|---|---|

## Single arm lifts

| | |
|---|---|
| **Setup** | Standing, feet wide apart, holding band under left foot and in left hand |
| **Exhale** | Lift band upwards to side |
| **Inhale** | Relax |
| | Repeat 10 x |

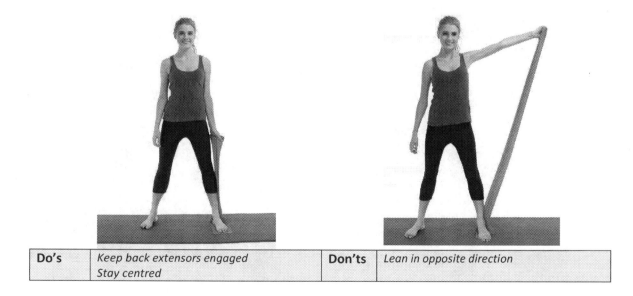

| Do's | Keep back extensors engaged<br>Stay centred | Don'ts | Lean in opposite direction |
|---|---|---|---|

## Arm lifts

**Setup**     Standing on band, feet hip width apart, holding band in both hands
**Exhale**    Bend arms and lift band in front
**Inhale**    Relax
                Repeat 10 x

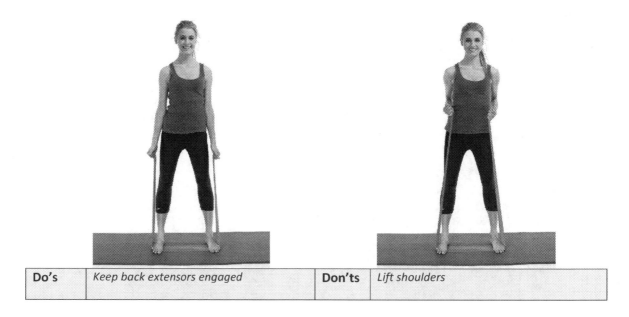

| Do's | Keep back extensors engaged | Don'ts | Lift shoulders |
|------|------------------------------|--------|----------------|

## Squats

**Setup**     Standing, feet hip width apart, band tied around legs under knees
**Exhale**    Bend and open knees
**Inhale**    Stretch legs
                Repeat 10 x and pulse 10 x

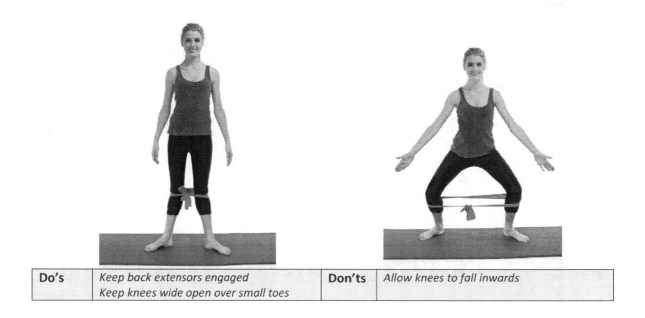

| Do's | Keep back extensors engaged<br>Keep knees wide open over small toes | Don'ts | Allow knees to fall inwards |
|------|---------------------------------------------------------------------|--------|------------------------------|

# *Abdominals*

## *Half roll down with leg lift*

**Setup**    Sitting, legs bent, band around one foot, holding band with both hands
**Exhale**    Roll down, straighten leg in line with knee
**Inhale**    Roll up
           Repeat 5 x

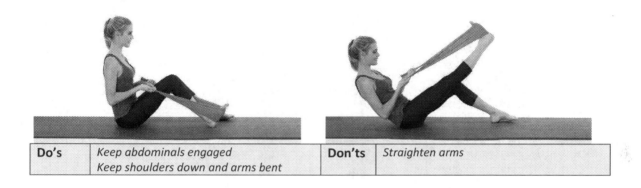

| Do's | Keep abdominals engaged<br>Keep shoulders down and arms bent | Don'ts | Straighten arms |
|------|-----------------------------------------------------------|--------|-----------------|

## *Teaser prep*

**Setup**    Sitting, legs bent, band around both feet, holding band with both hands
**Exhale**    Roll down and stretch legs
**Inhale**    Roll up
           Repeat 10 x

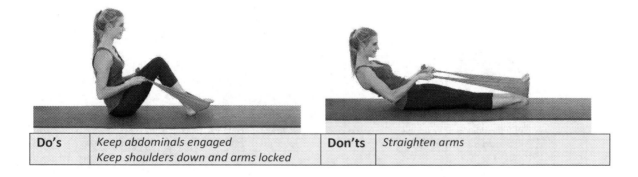

| Do's | Keep abdominals engaged<br>Keep shoulders down and arms locked | Don'ts | Straighten arms |
|------|--------------------------------------------------------------|--------|-----------------|

## Tabletop lift

**Setup**     Sitting, legs bent, band around both feet, holding band with both hands
**Exhale**    Lift legs to tabletop position
**Inhale**     Feet on floor
                Repeat 5 x

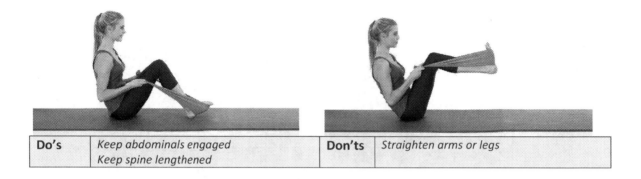

| Do's | Keep abdominals engaged<br>Keep spine lengthened | Don'ts | Straighten arms or legs |
| --- | --- | --- | --- |

## Teaser

**Setup**     Sitting, legs bent, band around both feet, holding band with both hands
**Exhale**    Stretch legs into V position
**Inhale**     Feet on floor
                Repeat 5 x

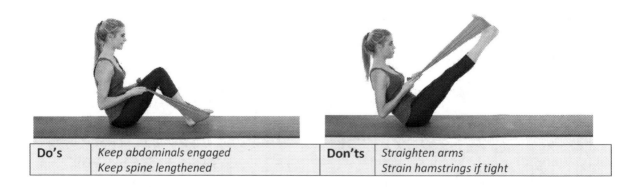

| Do's | Keep abdominals engaged<br>Keep spine lengthened | Don'ts | Straighten arms<br>Strain hamstrings if tight |
| --- | --- | --- | --- |

## Corkscrew prep

**Setup**   Lying supine, legs 90 degrees, band around feet, holding band with both hands
**Exhale**  Circle legs
**Inhale**  Legs back to start position
            Repeat 10 x alternating direction

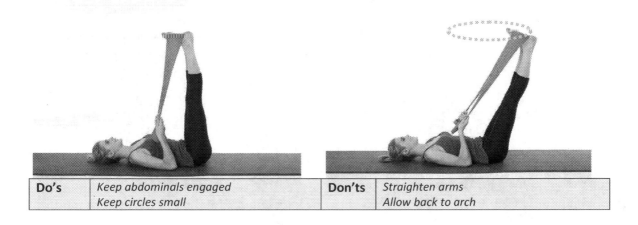

| Do's | Keep abdominals engaged<br>Keep circles small | Don'ts | Straighten arms<br>Allow back to arch |
|---|---|---|---|

## Legs side to side

**Setup**   Lying supine, legs 90 degrees, band around feet, holding band with both hands
**Exhale**  Drop legs to side
**Inhale**  Legs back to start position
            Repeat 10 x alternating sides

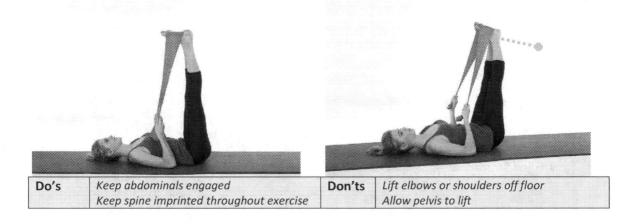

| Do's | Keep abdominals engaged<br>Keep spine imprinted throughout exercise | Don'ts | Lift elbows or shoulders off floor<br>Allow pelvis to lift |
|---|---|---|---|

# *Thighs and Butt*

## *Leg openings*

**Setup**   Lying supine, legs 90 degrees, band tied around ankles, palms on floor
**Exhale**  Open legs
**Inhale**  Relax
          Repeat 10 x pulse 10 x

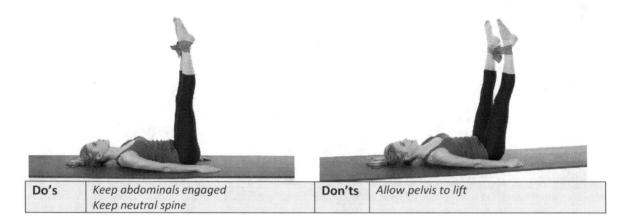

| Do's | Keep abdominals engaged <br> Keep neutral spine | Don'ts | Allow pelvis to lift |
|------|------------------------------------------------|--------|----------------------|

## *Leg lifts*

**Setup**   Lying on side, band tied around ankles
**Exhale**  Lift leg to hip height
**Inhale**  Relax
          Repeat 10 x pulse 10 x

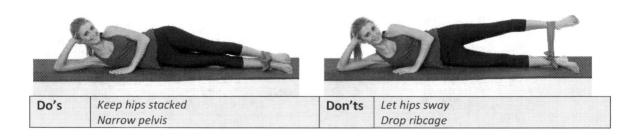

| Do's | Keep hips stacked <br> Narrow pelvis | Don'ts | Let hips sway <br> Drop ribcage |
|------|--------------------------------------|--------|---------------------------------|

## Sitting leg lifts

**Setup**    Sitting, legs straight, ankles crossed, hands at back, band tied around ankles
**Exhale**   Lift top leg up
**Inhale**   Relax
              Repeat 10 x change legs and repeat

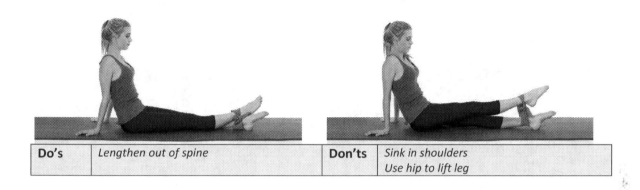

| Do's | Lengthen out of spine | Don'ts | Sink in shoulders<br>Use hip to lift leg |
|------|------------------------|--------|------------------------------------------|

## Side lying leg lifts

**Setup**    Lying on side, band tied around one foot, holding stretched band in one hand at sternum
**Exhale**   Lift leg to slightly higher than hip height
**Inhale**   Lower
              Repeat 10 x

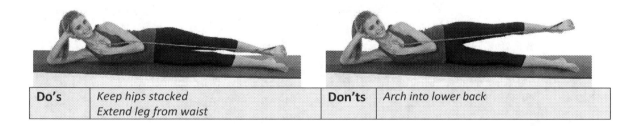

| Do's | Keep hips stacked<br>Extend leg from waist | Don'ts | Arch into lower back |
|------|---------------------------------------------|--------|----------------------|

## Doggie kick

**Setup**   Kneeling, one leg straight, band tied around foot, holding band in one hand
**Exhale**  Lift leg to hip height
**Inhale**  Back to start position
            Repeat 10 x

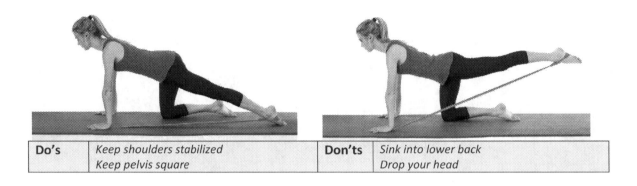

| Do's | Keep shoulders stabilized<br>Keep pelvis square | Don'ts | Sink into lower back<br>Drop your head |
|------|------------------------------------------------|--------|----------------------------------------|

## Leg circles

**Setup**   Lying supine, elbows on floor, band around one foot, holding band in both hands
**Exhale**  Circle leg
**Inhale**  Leg at 90 degrees
            Repeat 10 x clockwise and 10 x anti clockwise

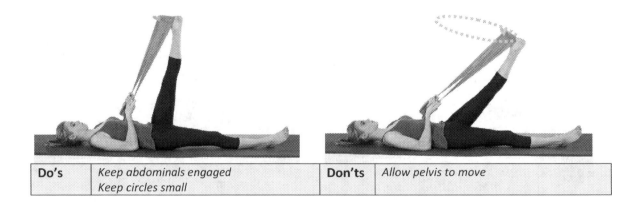

| Do's | Keep abdominals engaged<br>Keep circles small | Don'ts | Allow pelvis to move |
|------|-----------------------------------------------|--------|----------------------|

# Back Exercises

## Open legs

**Setup**    Lying prone, legs straight, band tied around ankles, chin on hands
**Exhale**    Open legs wide
**Inhale**    Legs together
        Repeat 5 x

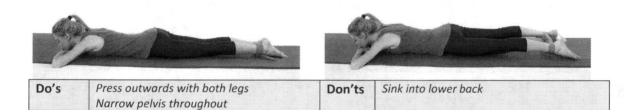

| Do's | Press outwards with both legs<br>Narrow pelvis throughout | Don'ts | Sink into lower back |
|------|----------------------------------------------------------|--------|----------------------|

## Star fish

**Setup**    Lying prone, legs straight, band tied around ankles, chin on hands
**Exhale**    Lift torso, open arms and legs wide, look in your mirror
**Inhale**    Legs together, fold hands under chin
        Repeat 10 x

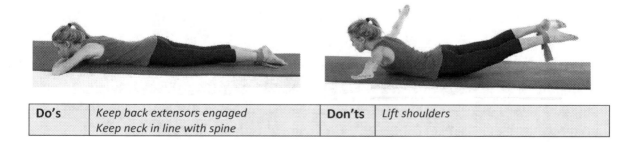

| Do's | Keep back extensors engaged<br>Keep neck in line with spine | Don'ts | Lift shoulders |
|------|-------------------------------------------------------------|--------|----------------|

# Spinal Rolls

## Roll over sitting

**Setup**   Sitting upright, legs straight, band around feet, holding band in both hands
**Exhale**  Roll back, stretch legs parallel to floor, press elbows into floor
**Inhale**  Roll up, stretch legs forward
            Repeat 5 x

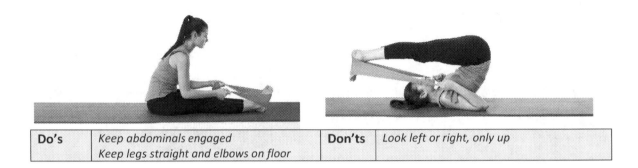

| Do's | Keep abdominals engaged<br>Keep legs straight and elbows on floor | Don'ts | Look left or right, only up |
|------|---|---|---|

## Roll over lying

**Setup**   Lying supine, legs 45 degrees, band around feet, holding band in both hands
**Exhale**  Pull legs over head, touch toes to floor, press elbows into floor
**Inhale**  Roll back slowly, legs back to 45 degrees
            Repeat 5 x

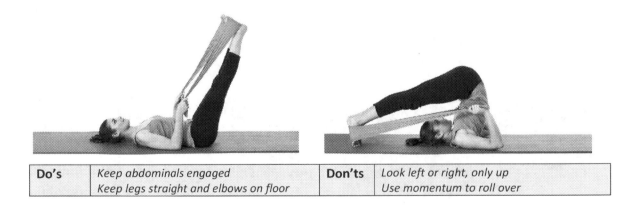

| Do's | Keep abdominals engaged<br>Keep legs straight and elbows on floor | Don'ts | Look left or right, only up<br>Use momentum to roll over |
|------|---|---|---|

A body free from nervous tension and

fatigue is the ideal shelter provided by

nature for housing a well balanced mind,

fully capable of successfully meeting the

complex problems of modern living.


Joseph Pilates

# Foam Roller

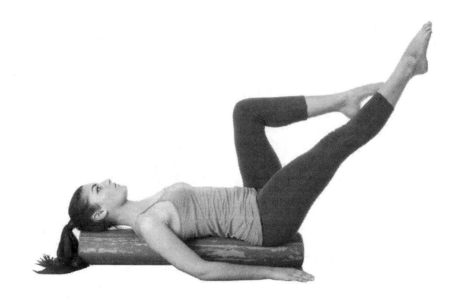

*Pilates is designed to give you suppleness,
natural grace and skill that will be
unmistakably reflected in the way
you walk, play and work*

*Joseph Pilates*

## *Why exercise with the foam roller?*

The foam roller will give you wonderful support for your back and spine. It will increase your ...

- ✓ Core stability
- ✓ Joint mobility
- ✓ Flexibility
- ✓ Strength
- ✓ Balance
- ✓ Suppleness

# *Warming Up*

## *Spinal stretch*

| | |
|---|---|
| **Setup** | Sitting on bent legs, roller in front, hands resting on roller |
| **Exhale** | Roll roller forward |
| **Inhale** | Roll roller backward |
| | Repeat 5 x |

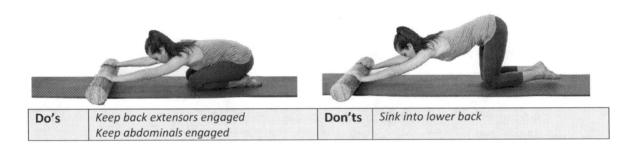

| Do's | Keep back extensors engaged<br>Keep abdominals engaged | Don'ts | Sink into lower back |
|---|---|---|---|

## *Shoulder stretch*

| | |
|---|---|
| **Setup** | Kneeling, hands resting on roller in line with shoulders |
| **Exhale** | Roll roller forward |
| **Inhale** | Roll roller backward |
| | Repeat 5 x |

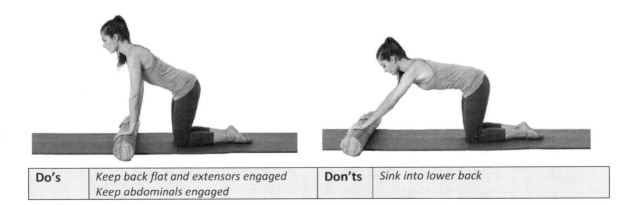

| Do's | Keep back flat and extensors engaged<br>Keep abdominals engaged | Don'ts | Sink into lower back |
|---|---|---|---|

# *Abdominals*

## *Single leg lifts*

**Setup**    Sitting, legs bent, roller under shoulder blades, arms stretched forward
**Inhale**   Bend leg towards chest
**Exhale**   Stretch leg to just above floor
**Inhale**   Bend leg towards chest
            Repeat 10 x

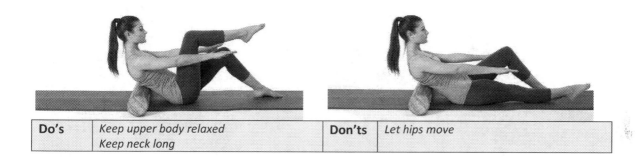

| Do's | Keep upper body relaxed<br>Keep neck long | Don'ts | Let hips move |
|------|---------|--------|--------|

## *Single leg bicycle*

**Setup**    Sitting, legs bent, roller under shoulder blades, palms on floor
**Inhale**   Bend and lift leg 90 degrees, point toe
**Exhale**   Flex foot and lower leg straight to floor
            Repeat 10x

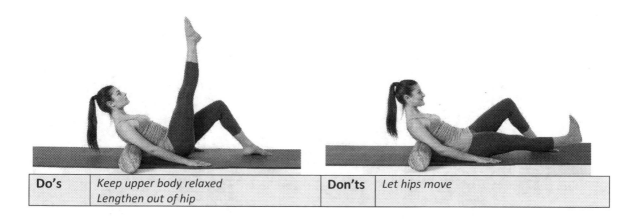

| Do's | Keep upper body relaxed<br>Lengthen out of hip | Don'ts | Let hips move |
|------|---------|--------|--------|

## Legs in V position

**Setup**   Sitting, legs bent, roller under shoulder blades, palms on floor
**Exhale**  Lift legs up to V position and open legs
**Inhale**  Legs together bend to touch floor
            Repeat 10 x

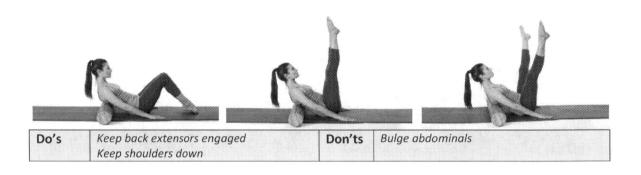

| Do's | Keep back extensors engaged<br>Keep shoulders down | Don'ts | Bulge abdominals |
|------|----------------------------------------------------|--------|------------------|

## Legs in tabletop

**Setup**   Sitting, legs bent, roller at lower back
**Exhale**  Lift legs up to tabletop
**Inhale**  Legs down to floor
            Repeat 10 x

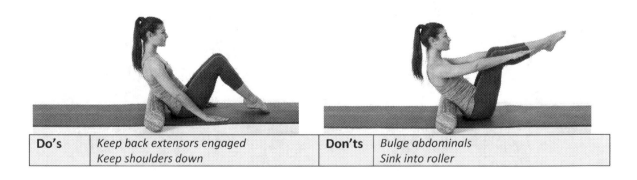

| Do's | Keep back extensors engaged<br>Keep shoulders down | Don'ts | Bulge abdominals<br>Sink into roller |
|------|----------------------------------------------------|--------|--------------------------------------|

## Single leg stretch

**Setup**    Lying supine on roller, legs in tabletop, palms on floor
**Exhale**   Stretch left leg
**Inhale**   Back to tabletop
            Repeat 10 x alternating legs

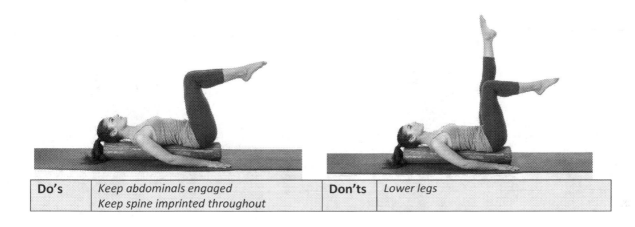

| Do's | Keep abdominals engaged<br>Keep spine imprinted throughout | Don'ts | Lower legs |
|------|---------------------------------------------------------|--------|-----------|

## Toe taps

**Setup**    Lying supine on roller, legs in tabletop, palms on floor
**Exhale**   Tap toe of left foot on floor 2 x
**Inhale**   Back to tabletop
            Repeat 10 x alternating legs

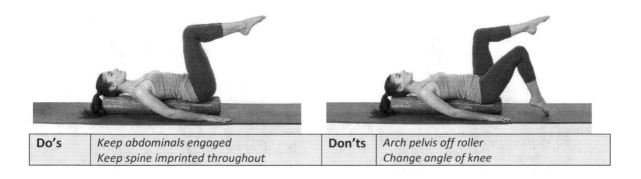

| Do's | Keep abdominals engaged<br>Keep spine imprinted throughout | Don'ts | Arch pelvis off roller<br>Change angle of knee |
|------|---------------------------------------------------------|--------|------------------------------------------------|

## Leg extensions

**Setup**     Lying supine on roller, legs in tabletop, palms on floor
**Exhale**    Stretch single leg to 45 degree angle
**Inhale**    Change legs
                Repeat 10 x alternating legs

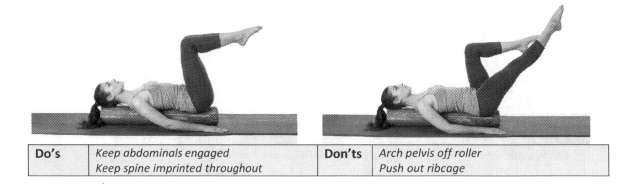

| **Do's** | *Keep abdominals engaged* | **Don'ts** | *Arch pelvis off roller* |
|---|---|---|---|
| | *Keep spine imprinted throughout* | | *Push out ribcage* |

## Double leg stretch

**Setup**     Lying supine on roller, legs in tabletop, palms on floor
**Exhale**    Stretch both legs to 45 degrees
**Inhale**    Back to tabletop
                Repeat 5 x

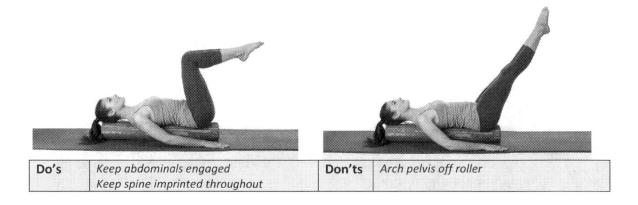

| **Do's** | *Keep abdominals engaged* | **Don'ts** | *Arch pelvis off roller* |
|---|---|---|---|
| | *Keep spine imprinted throughout* | | |

## Roll down

| | |
|---|---|
| **Setup** | Sitting on edge of roller, legs bent, arms stretched forward |
| **Exhale** | Roll back to lie on roller, circle arms backwards in full circle |
| **Inhale** | Roll up |
| | Repeat 10 x |

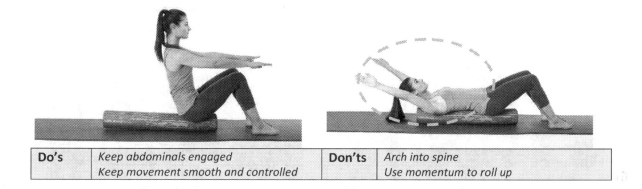

| Do's | Keep abdominals engaged<br>Keep movement smooth and controlled | Don'ts | Arch into spine<br>Use momentum to roll up |
|---|---|---|---|

## Knees off

| | |
|---|---|
| **Setup** | Kneeling, hands resting on roller in line with shoulders |
| **Exhale** | Push away from roller, lift knees just off the floor |
| **Inhale** | Knees on floor |
| | Repeat 10 x |

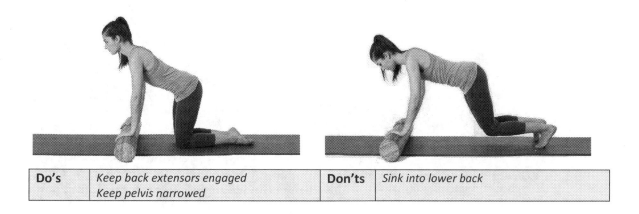

| Do's | Keep back extensors engaged<br>Keep pelvis narrowed | Don'ts | Sink into lower back |
|---|---|---|---|

# *Strengthening*

## *Back support prep*

| | |
|---|---|
| **Setup** | Sitting, legs bent, feet on roller, arms at back for support |
| **Exhale** | Lift hips into tabletop position |
| **Inhale** | Sit down |
| | Repeat 5 x |

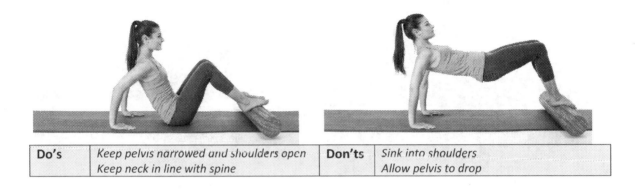

| Do's | Keep pelvis narrowed and shoulders open<br>Keep neck in line with spine | Don'ts | Sink into shoulders<br>Allow pelvis to drop |
|---|---|---|---|

## *Back support with leg extension*

| | |
|---|---|
| **Setup** | Sitting, legs bent, feet on roller, arms at back for support |
| **Exhale** | Lift hips up and stretch one leg upwards |
| **Inhale** | Down to floor |
| | Repeat 10 x alternating legs |

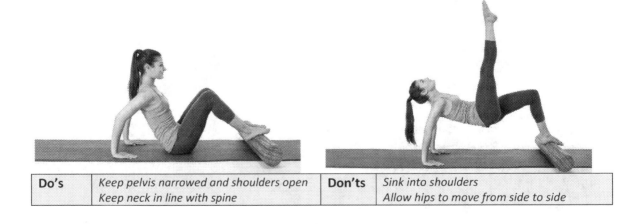

| Do's | Keep pelvis narrowed and shoulders open<br>Keep neck in line with spine | Don'ts | Sink into shoulders<br>Allow hips to move from side to side |
|---|---|---|---|

## Pelvic curl

| | |
|---|---|
| **Setup** | Lying supine, legs bent, feet on roller, palms on floor |
| **Exhale** | Roll spine off floor |
| **Inhale** | Roll back to starting position |
| | Repeat 10 x |

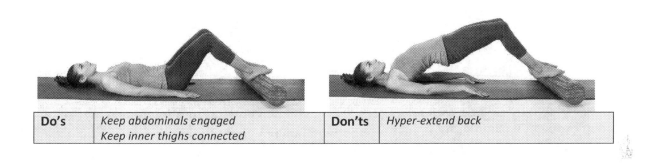

| **Do's** | Keep abdominals engaged<br>Keep inner thighs connected | **Don'ts** | Hyper-extend back |
|---|---|---|---|

## Pelvic curl with leg extensions

| | |
|---|---|
| **Setup** | Lying supine, legs bent, feet on roller, palms on floor |
| **Inhale** | Roll spine off floor |
| **Exhale** | Roll roller forwards with feet |
| **Inhale** | Roll roller backwards with feet, hips lifted |
| | Repeat 10 x |

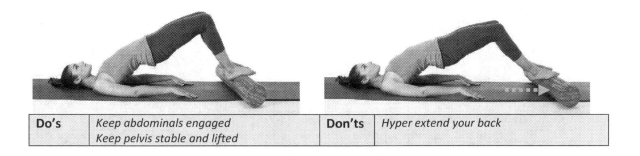

| **Do's** | Keep abdominals engaged<br>Keep pelvis stable and lifted | **Don'ts** | Hyper extend your back |
|---|---|---|---|

# Side Exercises

## Knee bend

**Setup**    Lying on elbow, roller under ribcage, top leg hip height
**Exhale**   Bend leg backwards, keeping knees in line
**Inhale**    Stretch leg out to starting position
            Repeat 10 x

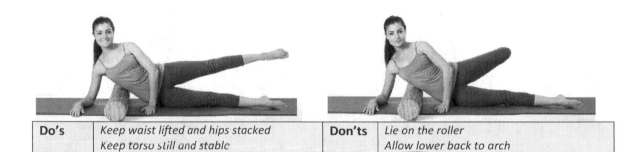

| Do's | Keep waist lifted and hips stacked<br>Keep torso still and stable | Don'ts | Lie on the roller<br>Allow lower back to arch |
|------|------------------------------------------------------------------|--------|-----------------------------------------------|

## Leg lift

**Setup**    Lying on elbow, roller under ribcage, legs straight
**Exhale**   Lift leg to hip height
**Inhale**    Lower leg to starting position
            Repeat 10 x

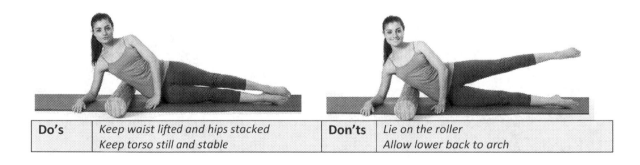

| Do's | Keep waist lifted and hips stacked<br>Keep torso still and stable | Don'ts | Lie on the roller<br>Allow lower back to arch |
|------|------------------------------------------------------------------|--------|-----------------------------------------------|

# *Back Exercises*

## *Swan dive prep*

| | |
|---|---|
| **Setup** | Lying prone, roller under pelvis, hands under shoulders |
| **Exhale** | Push up with arms |
| **Inhale** | Relax |
| | Repeat 5 x |

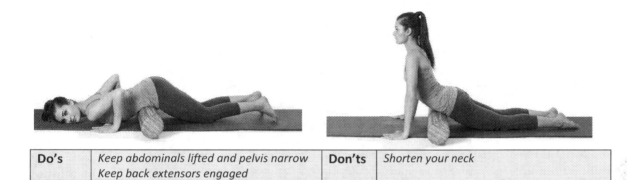

| Do's | Keep abdominals lifted and pelvis narrow<br>Keep back extensors engaged | Don'ts | Shorten your neck |
|---|---|---|---|

## *Single leg lift*

| | |
|---|---|
| **Setup** | Lying prone, roller under pelvis, hands under chin |
| **Exhale** | Lift leg upwards |
| **Inhale** | Down to start position |
| | Repeat 10 x alternating legs |
| | |
| | Repeat exercise lifting both legs |

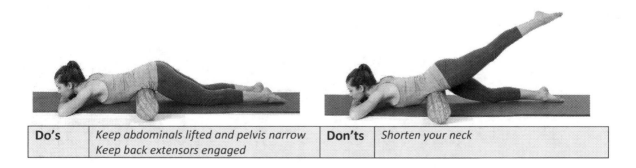

| Do's | Keep abdominals lifted and pelvis narrow<br>Keep back extensors engaged | Don'ts | Shorten your neck |
|---|---|---|---|

# The Pole

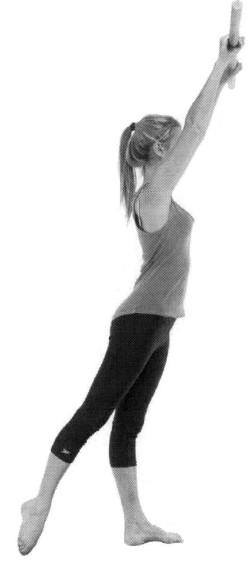

*A man is as young
as his spinal column*

Joseph Pilates

## *Why exercise with a Pole?*

The Pole is a very versatile and effective piece of exercise equipment that takes up virtually no space and will enhance every exercise you do.
It will …

- ✓ Improve your body alignment

- ✓ Improve your sense of balance

- ✓ Improve your suppleness

- ✓ Help you stretch even more

- ✓ Strengthen your body as a whole

*Enjoy every movement and stretch that you do with the Pole!*

---

The Pole used for the exercises is a wooden curtain rod
1,5 m (5 ft) long and 33 mm (1.25 in) diameter.

---

# Warming Up

## Arm reach

| | |
|---|---|
| **Setup** | Standing, feet hip width apart, holding pole with both hands |
| **Exhale** | Lift arms above head |
| **Inhale** | Lower arms |
| | Repeat 10 x |

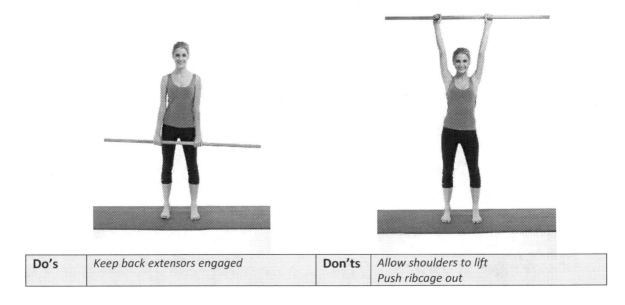

| **Do's** | Keep back extensors engaged | **Don'ts** | Allow shoulders to lift<br>Push ribcage out |
|---|---|---|---|

## Single arm lift

| | |
|---|---|
| **Setup** | Standing, feet hip width apart, holding pole with one hand |
| **Exhale** | Lift arm to shoulder height |
| **Inhale** | Lower arm |
| | Repeat 10 x each arm |

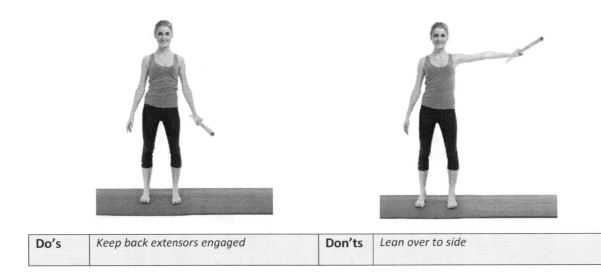

| **Do's** | Keep back extensors engaged | **Don'ts** | Lean over to side |
|---|---|---|---|

## Squat with shoulder press

**Setup**   Standing, feet hip width apart, pole resting on shoulders
**Exhale**  Bend knees, stretch arms above head
**Inhale**  Straighten legs, lower arms
            Repeat 10 x

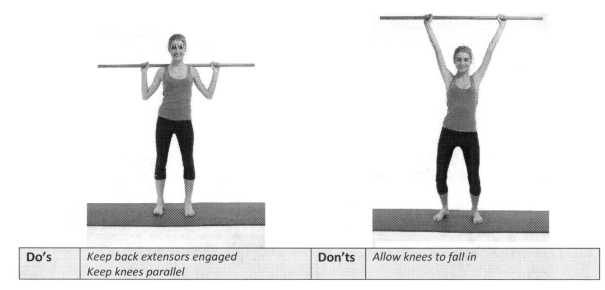

| Do's | Keep back extensors engaged<br>Keep knees parallel | Don'ts | Allow knees to fall in |
|------|---------------------------------------------------|--------|------------------------|

## Squat with leg lift

**Setup**   Standing, feet hip width apart, pole resting on shoulders
**Inhale**  Bend knees
**Exhale**  Move weight to left side, lift right leg off floor
**Inhale**  Back to centre, knees stay bent
**Exhale**  Move weight to right side, lift left leg off floor
            Repeat 10 x

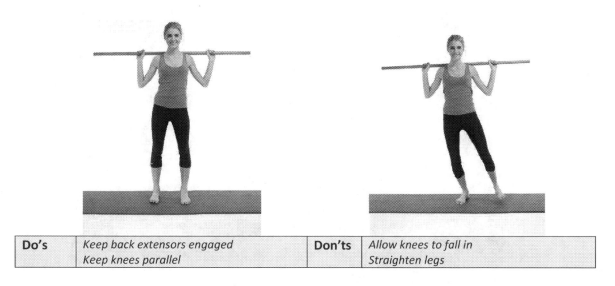

| Do's | Keep back extensors engaged<br>Keep knees parallel | Don'ts | Allow knees to fall in<br>Straighten legs |
|------|---------------------------------------------------|--------|-------------------------------------------|

## Forward lunge with shoulder press

**Setup**    Standing, one foot in front, foot turned out, pole resting on shoulders
**Exhale**   Bend both knees, stretch arms above head
**Inhale**    Straighten legs, lower pole
            Repeat 5 x left foot in front, 5 x right foot in front

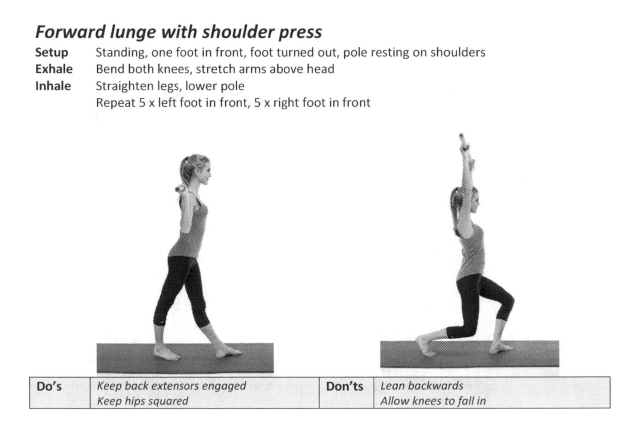

| Do's | Keep back extensors engaged<br>Keep hips squared | Don'ts | Lean backwards<br>Allow knees to fall in |
| --- | --- | --- | --- |

## Forward reach with hinge

**Setup**    Standing, one foot in front, foot turned out, holding pole in front
**Exhale**   Bend front knee, lean forward to 45 degrees, stretch arms in line with ears
**Inhale**    Straighten legs, lower pole
            Repeat 5 x left foot in front, 5 x right foot in front

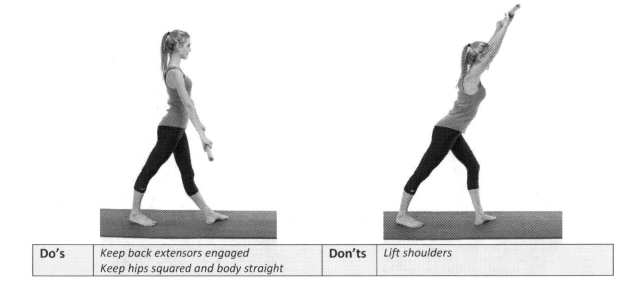

| Do's | Keep back extensors engaged<br>Keep hips squared and body straight | Don'ts | Lift shoulders |
| --- | --- | --- | --- |

## Knee lift with rotation

| | |
|---|---|
| **Setup** | Standing, feet together, holding pole in front |
| **Inhale** | Lift knee in front, arms at shoulder height |
| **Exhale** | Turn torso over leg |
| **Inhale** | Feet together, lower pole |
| | Repeat 10 x alternating sides |

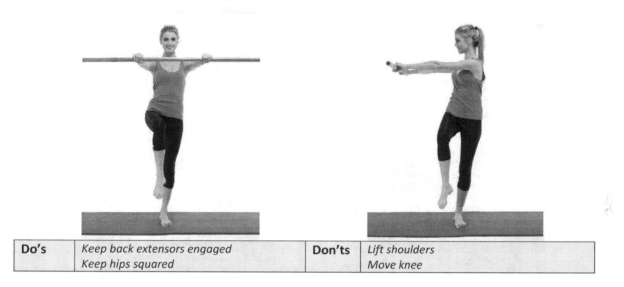

| Do's | Keep back extensors engaged<br>Keep hips squared | Don'ts | Lift shoulders<br>Move knee |
|---|---|---|---|

## Back leg lift

| | |
|---|---|
| **Setup** | Standing, one foot in front and turned out, holding pole in front |
| **Exhale** | Point toe at back, left leg off floor, stretch arms in line with ears |
| **Inhale** | Lower leg, press heel into the floor and lower pole |
| | Repeat 10 x |

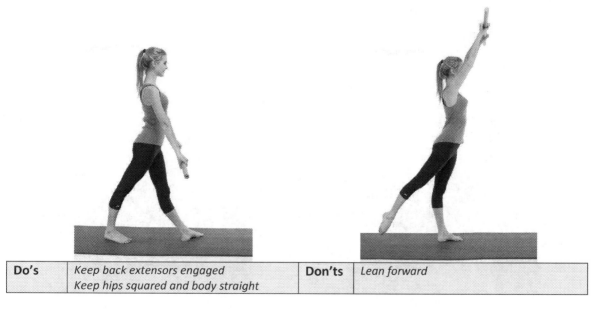

| Do's | Keep back extensors engaged<br>Keep hips squared and body straight | Don'ts | Lean forward |
|---|---|---|---|

# Abdominals

## Leg extension with rotation

**Setup**   Sitting upright, legs bent, holding pole in front with both hands
**Exhale**   Lift left leg in line with knee, twist torso over leg to left side
**Inhale**   Back to start position
Repeat 10 x alternating sides

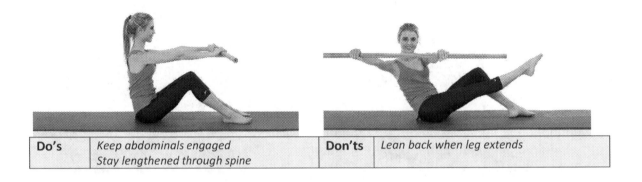

| **Do's** | Keep abdominals engaged<br>Stay lengthened through spine | **Don'ts** | Lean back when leg extends |
|---|---|---|---|

## Half roll down oblique

**Setup**   Sitting upright, legs straight, holding pole overhead with both hands
**Exhale**   Lean back 45 degrees, rotate torso to side
**Inhale**   Back to start position
Repeat 10 x alternating sides

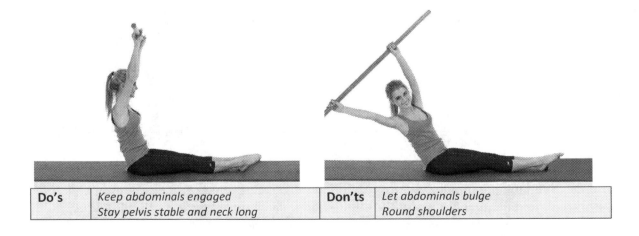

| **Do's** | Keep abdominals engaged<br>Stay pelvis stable and neck long | **Don'ts** | Let abdominals bulge<br>Round shoulders |
|---|---|---|---|

## Single leg roll up

**Setup**    Lying supine, legs bent, holding pole overhead on floor
**Exhale**   Roll up to sitting position, stretch leg, touch pole on leg
**Inhale**   Roll down to start position
             Repeat 10 x alternating legs

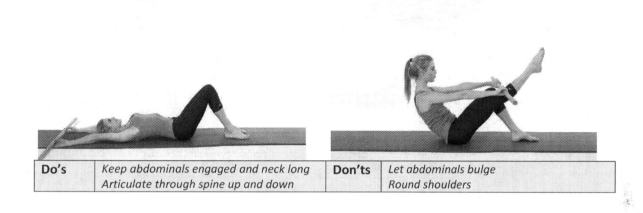

| Do's | Keep abdominals engaged and neck long | Don'ts | Let abdominals bulge |
|------|----------------------------------------|--------|----------------------|
|      | *Articulate through spine up and down* |        | *Round shoulders*    |

## Double leg stretch

**Setup**    Lying supine, legs bent, holding pole under knees
**Exhale**   Lift shoulders, stretch legs and arms
**Inhale**   Back to start position
             Repeat 10 x

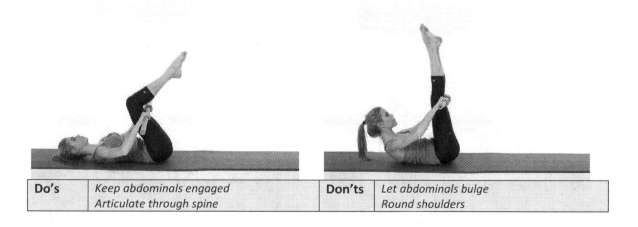

| Do's | Keep abdominals engaged | Don'ts | Let abdominals bulge |
|------|--------------------------|--------|----------------------|
|      | *Articulate through spine* |      | *Round shoulders*    |

## Double leg lift

**Setup**     Sitting upright, legs bent, holding pole under knees
**Exhale**    Lift legs into tabletop position
**Inhale**     Back to start position
            Repeat 5 x

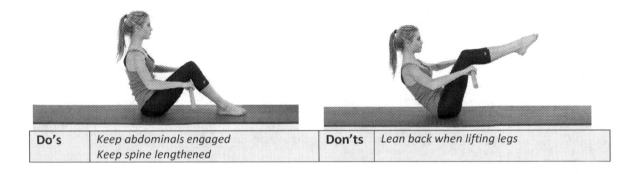

| Do's | Keep abdominals engaged<br>Keep spine lengthened | Don'ts | Lean back when lifting legs |
|------|--------------------------------------------------|--------|-----------------------------|

## Teaser prep

**Setup**     Sitting upright, legs bent, holding pole under knees
**Exhale**    Stretch legs into V position
**Inhale**     Back to start position
            Repeat 5 x

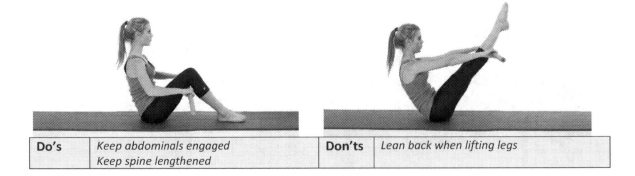

| Do's | Keep abdominals engaged<br>Keep spine lengthened | Don'ts | Lean back when lifting legs |
|------|--------------------------------------------------|--------|-----------------------------|

# Side Exercises

## Side lying leg lift

**Setup**　　Lying on side, pole resting on left foot, holding pole in left hand
**Exhale**　　Lift left leg slightly higher than hip height, foot flexed
**Inhale**　　Down to floor
　　　　　　Repeat 10 x, pulse 10 x

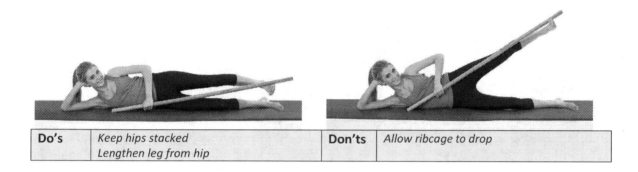

| Do's | Keep hips stacked<br>Lengthen leg from hip | Don'ts | Allow ribcage to drop |
|------|---------------------------------------------|--------|------------------------|

## Side lying inner thigh lift

**Setup**　　Lying on side, right leg bent, pole resting on left foot, holding pole in left hand
**Exhale**　　Lift body off floor, left leg to hip height, foot flexed
**Inhale**　　Down to floor
　　　　　　Repeat 10 x

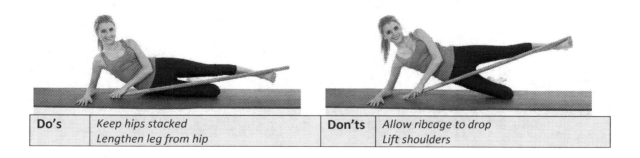

| Do's | Keep hips stacked<br>Lengthen leg from hip | Don'ts | Allow ribcage to drop<br>Lift shoulders |
|------|---------------------------------------------|--------|------------------------------------------|

# Back Exercises

## Chest expansion

**Setup**    Lying prone, holding pole at back with both hands
**Exhale**   Lift arms
**Inhale**   Relax
             Repeat 5 x

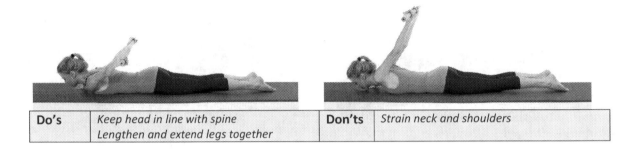

| Do's | Keep head in line with spine<br>Lengthen and extend legs together | Don'ts | Strain neck and shoulders |
| --- | --- | --- | --- |

## Swan dive

**Setup**    Lying prone, holding pole at back with both hands
**Exhale**   Lift arms and legs
**Inhale**   Relax
             Repeat 5 x

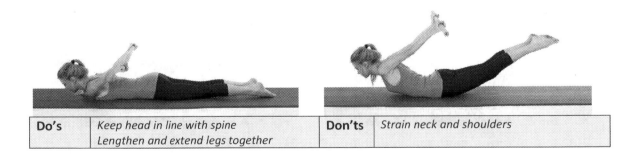

| Do's | Keep head in line with spine<br>Lengthen and extend legs together | Don'ts | Strain neck and shoulders |
| --- | --- | --- | --- |

# Spinal Rolls

## Rolling like a ball

| | |
|---|---|
| **Setup** | Sitting, pole under knees, holding pole with both hands |
| **Exhale** | Roll back, stretch legs parallel to floor |
| **Inhale** | Roll up, bend knees |
| | Repeat 5 x |

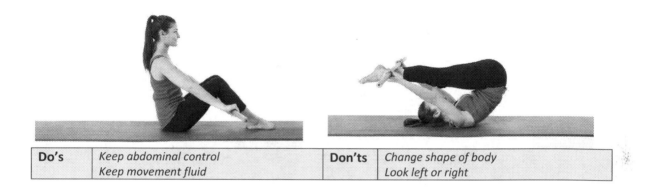

| Do's | Keep abdominal control<br>Keep movement fluid | Don'ts | Change shape of body<br>Look left or right |
|---|---|---|---|

## Roll over

| | |
|---|---|
| **Setup** | Lying supine, legs 90 degrees, pole behind legs, holding pole with both hands |
| **Exhale** | Pull legs over body until toes touch floor |
| **Inhale** | Back to start position |
| | Repeat 5 x |

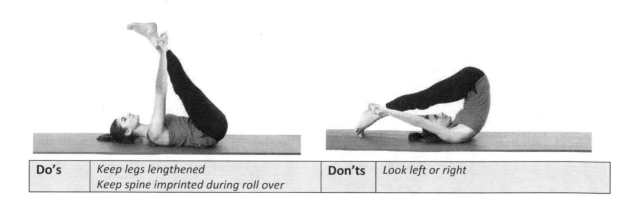

| Do's | Keep legs lengthened<br>Keep spine imprinted during roll over | Don'ts | Look left or right |
|---|---|---|---|

# Let's Stretch

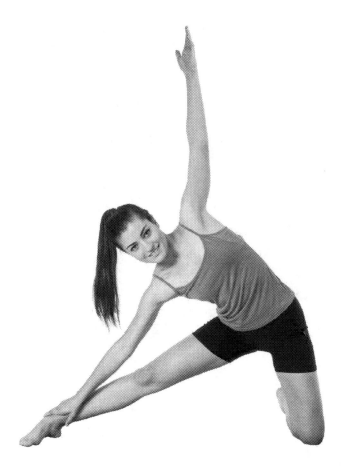

# *Why do we need to stretch?*

✓ Stretching improves mobility and flexibility and it will reduce your chances of injury.

✓ Stretching will counter tightness by lengthening your muscles and helping your joints maintain a natural range of motion.

✓ Stretching is an essential component of fitness as it enhances your quality of movement.

✓ Stretching can be a program on its own or as a cool down after exercising.

✓ Stretch only as far as it is comfortable for you.

Hold every stretch for 10 to 30 seconds and longer if you feel comfortable.
Always listen to your body and 'feel' your muscles.
Remember to warm up your muscles before you start stretching.
Warm muscles will minimize the risk of injuries.

# *Stretching*

## *Neck pull*

**Setup**  Standing, feet hip width apart, fingers interlaced behind your head
Pull your head forward
Lift head
Repeat

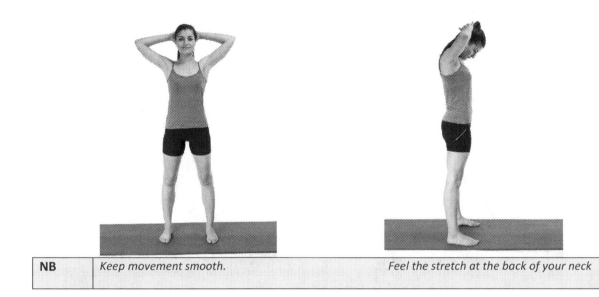

| NB | *Keep movement smooth.* | *Feel the stretch at the back of your neck* |
|----|-------------------------|---------------------------------------------|

## *Backward reach*

**Setup**  Standing, feet hip width apart, arms at sides
Swing arms up and lean backwards
Straighten body, lower arms
Repeat

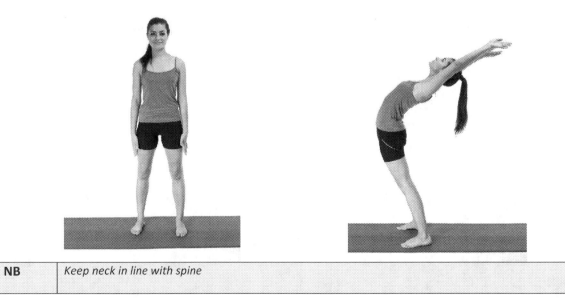

| NB | *Keep neck in line with spine* |
|----|--------------------------------|

## Arm pull

**Setup**     Standing, feet hip width apart
Stretch left arm across chest, pull left arm with right hand across chest
Relax
Repeat alternating sides

*Feel the stretch in your arm and shoulder*

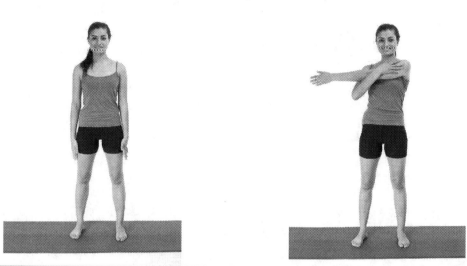

| NB | Keep torso facing forward | Keep arm across chest straight |
|----|---------------------------|-------------------------------|

## Overhead reach to side

**Setup**     Standing, feet hip width apart, arms above head, fingers interlaced, palms facing up.
Stretch arms up and bend into left side
Straighten body and bend into right side
Repeat alternating sides

*WOW feel those sides!*

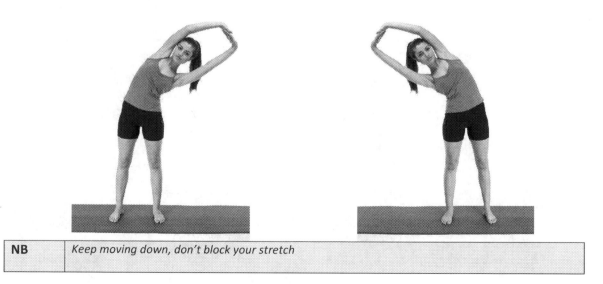

| NB | Keep moving down, don't block your stretch |
|----|--------------------------------------------|

## Pectoral stretch

**Setup**     Standing, feet hip width apart, fingers interlaced behind back
                    Lift arms at back and bend forward, pulling arms over body
                    Back to start position
                    Repeat

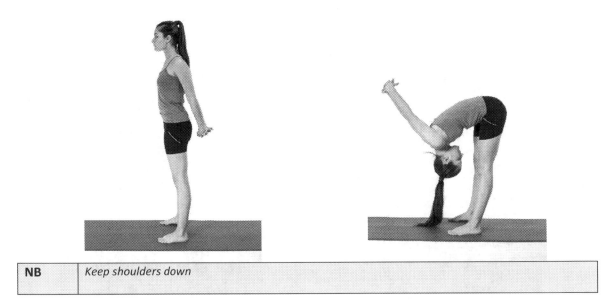

| NB | Keep shoulders down |
|----|---------------------|

## Overhead reach to side

**Setup**     Standing, feet together
                    Slide left hand down leg, bend leg slightly
                    Stretch right arm upwards
                    Repeat alternating sides

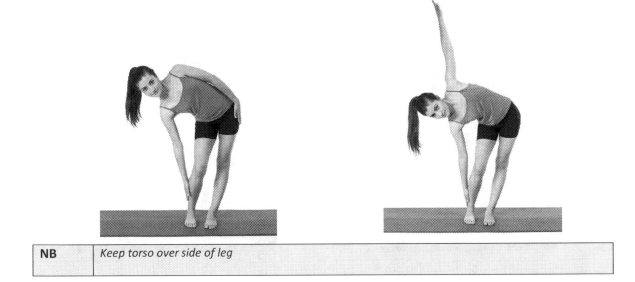

| NB | Keep torso over side of leg |
|----|-----------------------------|

## Standing stretch

**Setup**    Standing, feet wide apart, hands on floor
Bend right leg, right elbow on floor
Bend left leg, left elbow on floor
Repeat alternating sides

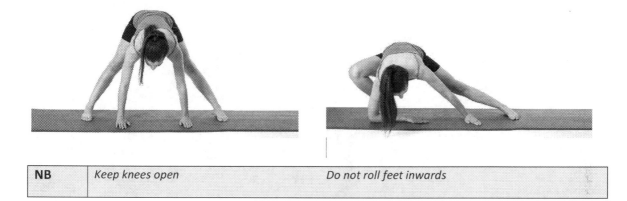

| NB | Keep knees open | Do not roll feet inwards |
|----|-----------------|--------------------------|

## Forward stretch

**Setup**    Standing, feet wide apart, hands on floor
Bend right leg, right hand on floor, stretch left arm in front
Bend left leg, left hand on floor, stretch right arm in front
Repeat alternating sides

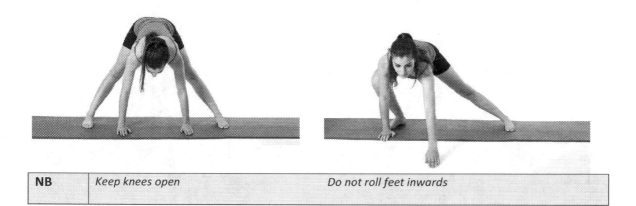

| NB | Keep knees open | Do not roll feet inwards |
|----|-----------------|--------------------------|

## *Hip flexor stretch*

**Setup**  Right leg bent at 90 degree angle, left leg behind, hands on floor in line with heel
Straighten left leg, push heel away from body
Hold stretch and relax
Repeat

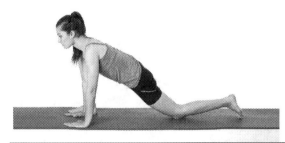 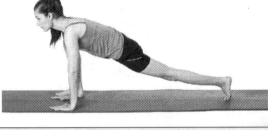

| NB | Keep hips facing forward | Do not allow knee to pass ankle |
|----|--------------------------|--------------------------------|

## *Kneeling side stretch*

**Setup**  Left knee on floor, right leg stretched to side
Slide right arm down on leg, stretch left arm into side bend and hold
Turn torso and stretch forward over straight leg, hold
Repeat

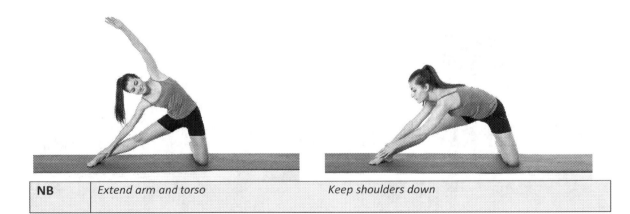

| NB | Extend arm and torso | Keep shoulders down |
|----|----------------------|---------------------|

## Kneeling fold down

**Setup**   Right leg bent, left knee on floor, right hand on floor in front of right foot
Go into side bend with left arm and hold
Place elbows in front on floor and hold
Repeat

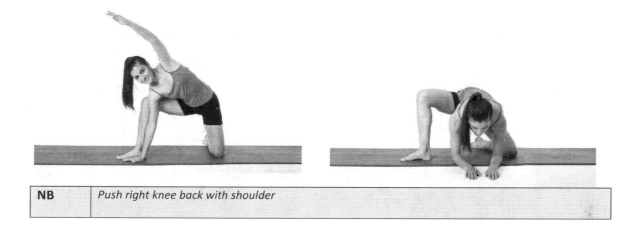

| NB | *Push right knee back with shoulder* | |
|----|--------------------------------------|--|

## Tendon stretch

**Setup**   Standing, feet together, knees bent slightly, chest on knees, hands holding ankles
Stretch legs, chest stays glued to knees
Release and repeat

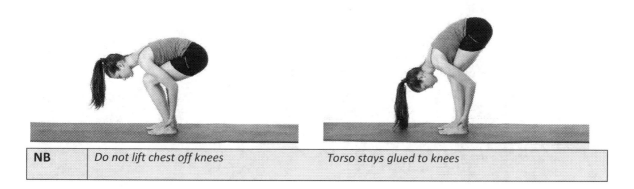

| NB | *Do not lift chest off knees* | *Torso stays glued to knees* |
|----|-------------------------------|------------------------------|

## Thigh stretch

**Setup**    Sitting on bent legs, hands at back on floor
Push hips up
Sit down
Repeat

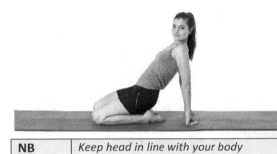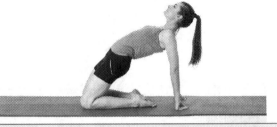

| NB | Keep head in line with your body | Lift up and push forward from your hips up towards your shoulders |
|----|----------------------------------|------------------------------------------------------------------|

## Overhead stretch

**Setup**    Sitting on bent legs, fingers interlaced at back
Bend forward, place head on floor, lift arms at back and bring over body
Straighten up  to start position
Repeat

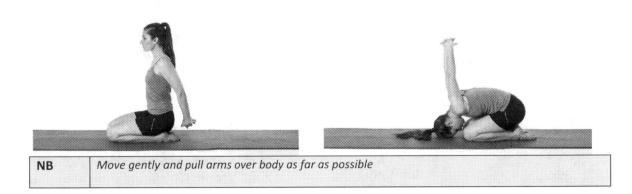

| NB | Move gently and pull arms over body as far as possible |
|----|--------------------------------------------------------|

## Wrist stretch

**Setup**     Kneeling, hands on floor, fingers facing knees
Lean back, feel the stretch in your wrists
Relax
Repeat

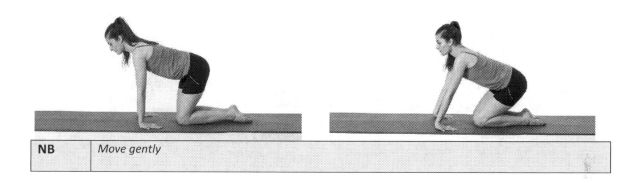

| NB | *Move gently* |
|----|---------------|

## Sitting spine twist

**Setup**     Sitting upright, legs straight, left hand holding right foot
Stretch right arm to back, bend left elbow onto knees, look at right arm
Repeat

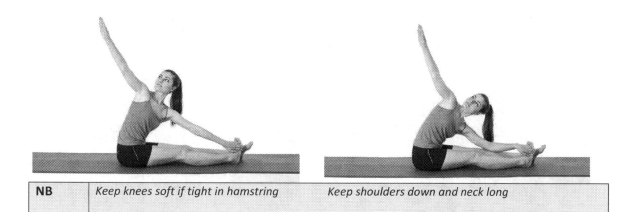

| NB | *Keep knees soft if tight in hamstring* | *Keep shoulders down and neck long* |
|----|----------------------------------------|-------------------------------------|

## Sitting side bend

**Setup**    Sitting upright, legs folded, ankles not crossed
Place right hand on floor, go into side bend to the right
Place left hand on floor, go into side bend to the left
Place hands on floor in centre and stretch forward
Fold feet opposite way and repeat

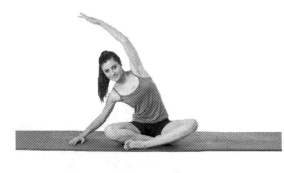
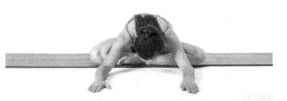

| NB | Extend arm and torso in side bend. | Extend arms and torso in forward bend |
|----|-----|-----|

## Legs crossed side bend

**Setup**    Sitting upright, left leg bent with right foot over left knee
Stretch left arm up into side bend
Stretch right arm up into side bend
Place both hands on floor in front an
Fold legs the opposite way and repeat

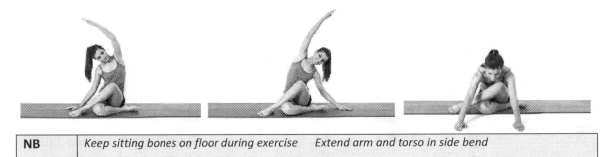

| NB | Keep sitting bones on floor during exercise | Extend arm and torso in side bend |
|----|-----|-----|

## Mermaid stretch

**Setup**     Sitting upright, both legs bent to left side
              Stretch right arm up into side bend
              Turn and place both hands on floor in line with hips
              Bend arms and touch chin on floor
              Stretch arms and look over right shoulder
              Repeat

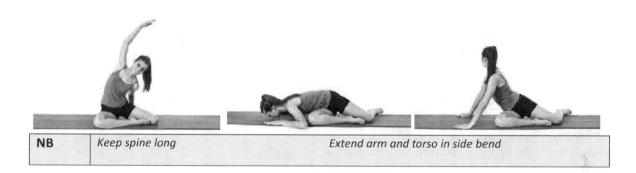

| NB | Keep spine long | Extend arm and torso in side bend |
|----|-----------------|-----------------------------------|

## Forward bend with sideways and backward stretch

**Setup**     Sitting upright, legs straight
              Stretch forward and touch toes
              Turn sideways, place hands on floor in line with hip, rest forehead on floor, heels on floor
              Repeat to opposite side

              Sit up, stretch forward and touch toes
              Turn around, place hands on floor in line with shoulders, rest forehead on floor
              Repeat to opposite side

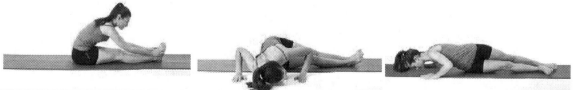

| Do's | Extend torso throughout exercise | Keep both heels on floor |
|------|----------------------------------|--------------------------|

# At the Barre

## Lower back and tendon stretch

**Setup**    Standing facing barre, holding barre with both hands, feet  wide apart
Stretch arms with flat back.  Feel as if you push your body through your arms
Hold
Straighten up, lean forward in a straight line

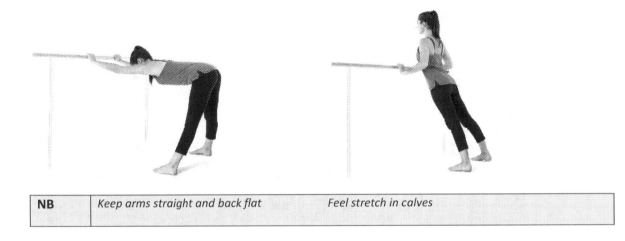

| NB | Keep arms straight and back flat | Feel stretch in calves |
|----|----------------------------------|------------------------|

## Backward lunge

**Setup**    Standing facing barre, holding  with both hands
Slide one leg far back keeping body upright, front knee at 90 degree angle
Repeat alternating legs

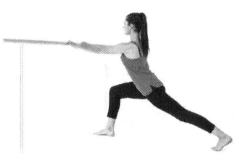

| NB | Keep spine long and knees squared | Push heel away from body |
|----|-----------------------------------|--------------------------|

## Side stretch

**Setup**    Standing close to barre, holding bar with one hand, feet together
Swing arm up into side bend, hang away from the  barre with a straight arm
Repeat

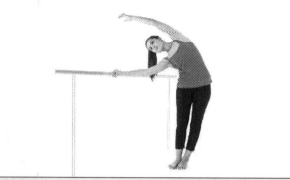

| NB | *Feel the stretch in your side* | *Hang away from barre* |
|----|----------------------------------|------------------------|

## Pectoral stretch

**Setup**    Standing with back towards barre, holding barre with both hands, feet together
Lean forward, pull away from barre
Release
Repeat

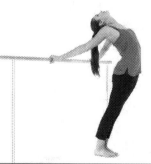

| NB | *Stretch arms and pull away from barre* | *Push forward with shoulders and hips* |
|----|------------------------------------------|----------------------------------------|

# Big Ball

## Sitting side bend

**Setup**  Sitting on ball, arms to sides
Lift left arm up into side bend.  Arm down
Lift right arm up into side bend.  Arm down
Repeat

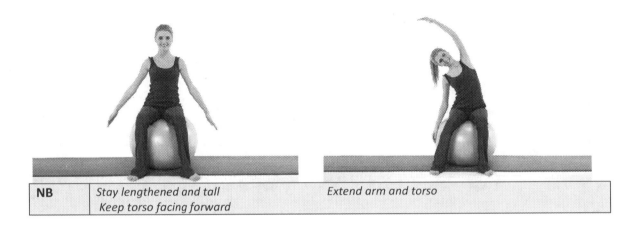

| NB | Stay lengthened and tall | Extend arm and torso |
|----|--------------------------|----------------------|
|    | Keep torso facing forward |                     |

## Arm reach

**Setup**  Sitting on ball, arms at back on ball
Push on ball with right hand, stand up and stretch left arm
Sit down on ball
Repeat  alternating sides

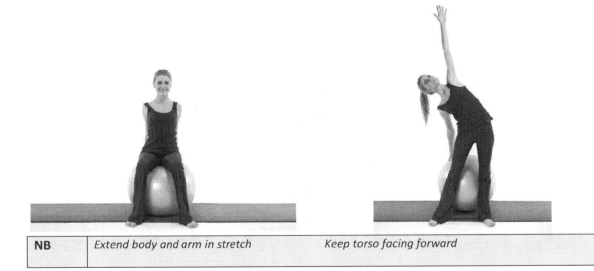

| NB | Extend body and arm in stretch | Keep torso facing forward |
|----|--------------------------------|---------------------------|

## Side bend

**Setup**     Standing, feet hip width apart, holding ball
                 Swing ball up into left side bend
                 Ball down
                 Swing ball up into right side bend
                 Repeat

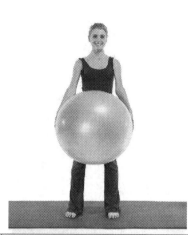 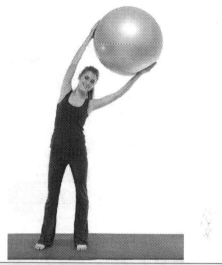

| NB | *Feel the stretch in your sides* | *Keep torso facing forward and arms extended* |
|----|----------------------------------|-----------------------------------------------|

## Standing spine stretch

**Setup**     Standing, feet wide apart, hands on ball in front
                 Roll ball forward, stretch out your back
                 Roll ball to left side and back to centre
                 Roll ball to right side and back to centre

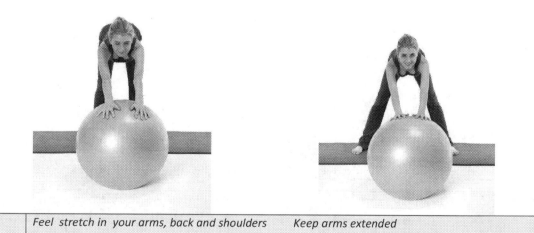

| NB | *Feel stretch in your arms, back and shoulders* | *Keep arms extended* |
|----|--------------------------------------------------|------------------------|

## Thigh stretch

**Setup**   Kneeling with lower back resting on ball
Push hips up
Relax
Repeat

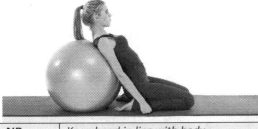 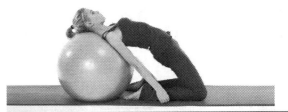

| NB | Keep head in line with body | Push hips up |
|----|------------------------------|--------------|

## Full body stretch

**Setup**   Lying with legs bent, head and shoulders supported on ball
Stretch legs, roll backwards over ball
Roll back to start position
Repeat

*WONDERFULL!*

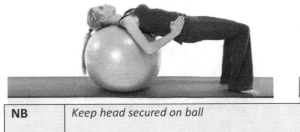 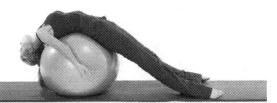

| NB | Keep head secured on ball | Keep both feet firmly on floor |
|----|----------------------------|--------------------------------|

## *Kneeling spine stretch*

**Setup**     Kneeling with both hands resting on ball, arms straight
              Roll ball forward, feel as if you are pushing your body through your arms
              Roll ball backwards
              Repeat

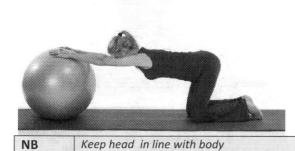
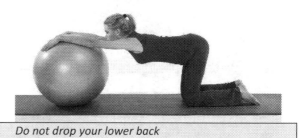

| NB | Keep head in line with body | Do not drop your lower back |
|----|------------------------------|------------------------------|

## *Shoulder stretch*

**Setup**     Sitting on bent legs, right hand resting on ball
              Roll ball over to left side, back of right hand in touch with ball
              Roll back to centre
              Repeat

*Feel the stretch in your arm and shoulder*

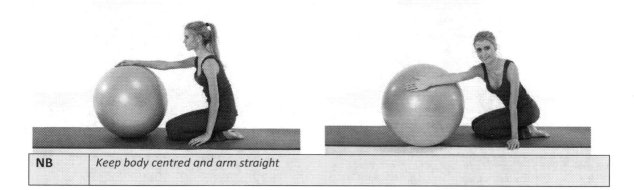

| NB | Keep body centred and arm straight |
|----|-------------------------------------|

## Side stretch

**Setup**     Kneeling on side of ball, one leg stretched to side, one hand on ball
Roll ball away, stretch arm over ball in side bend
Lift up and roll ball in
Repeat

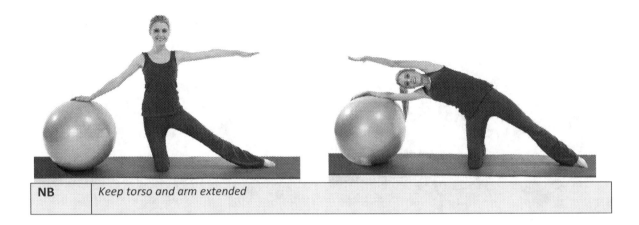

| NB | Keep torso and arm extended |
|----|------------------------------|

## Hip flexor stretch

**Setup**     Kneeling on one knee, hands on ball for balance and support
Stretch leg out at back
Relax knee to floor
Repeat

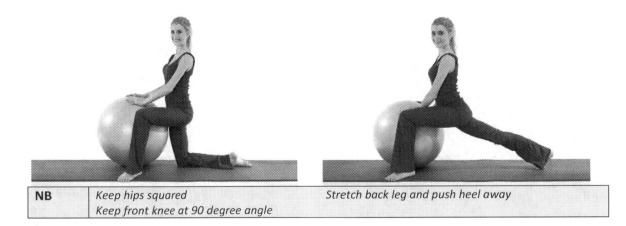

| NB | Keep hips squared<br>Keep front knee at 90 degree angle | Stretch back leg and push heel away |
|----|----------------------------------------------------------|--------------------------------------|

## Threading the needle

**Setup**   Kneeling with ball in front, both hands resting on ball
Push right arm through under torso
Change arms
Repeat

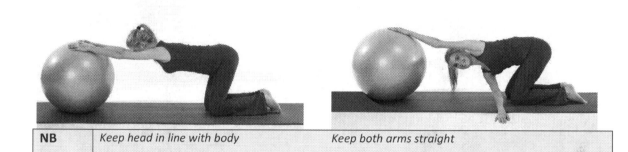

| NB | Keep head in line with body | Keep both arms straight |
|----|------------------------------|--------------------------|

## Hamstring stretch

**Setup**   Lying supine, legs bent, ball resting on right thigh, left leg draped over ball
Stretch left leg
Relax leg
Repeat

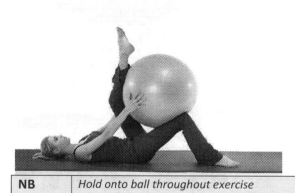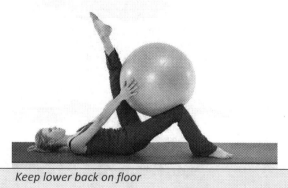

| NB | Hold onto ball throughout exercise | Keep lower back on floor |
|----|-------------------------------------|---------------------------|

# *Small Ball*

## *Spine twist*

**Setup**   Standing, feet hip width apart, holding ball in front at shoulder height
Rotate torso to right
Face front
Rotate torso to left

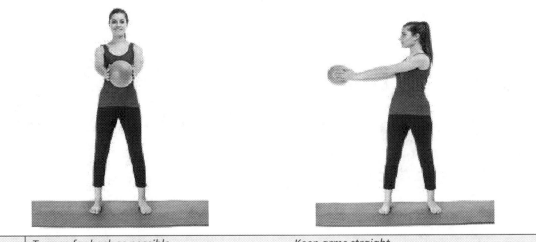

| NB | Turn as far back as possible | Keep arms straight |
|----|------------------------------|--------------------|

## *Shoulder stretch*

**Setup**   Standing, feet hip width apart, holding ball at back with both hands
Lift arms up
Lower arms
Repeat

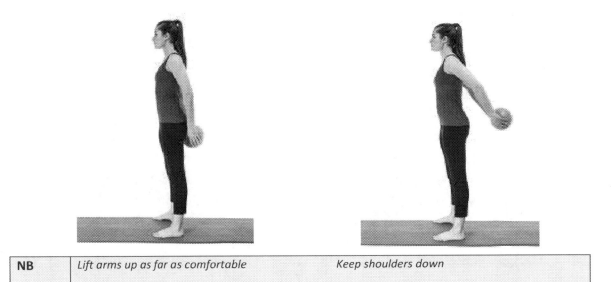

| NB | Lift arms up as far as comfortable | Keep shoulders down |
|----|------------------------------------|---------------------|

## Pectoral stretch

**Setup**    Standing, feet hip width apart, holding ball at back with both hands
Lift arms at back, bend forward bringing arms over body
Straighten body and lower arms
Repeat

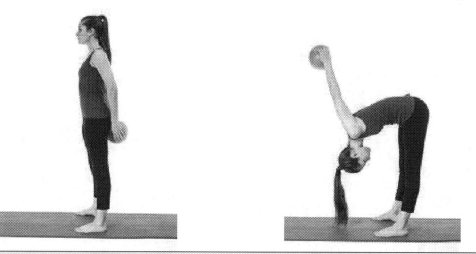

| NB | *Pull arms over body as far as comfortable* |
|----|---------------------------------------------|

## Side bend

**Setup**    Standing, feet hip width apart, holding ball in front at shoulder height
Swing arms into side bend
Lower arms to front
Repeat

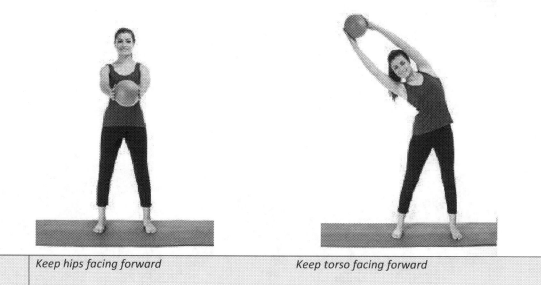

| NB | *Keep hips facing forward* | *Keep torso facing forward* |
|----|----------------------------|-----------------------------|

## *Side bend with bent legs*

**Setup**  Sit on floor with both legs bent to left side
Lift arms up and go into side bend
Place ball on floor and roll forward
Repeat

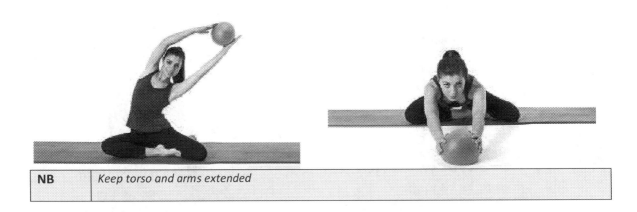

| NB | *Keep torso and arms extended* |
|----|--------------------------------|

## *Side bend with straight leg*

**Setup**  Sitting, right leg folded in, left leg stretched to side, holding ball in both hands
Lift arms upwards, go into side bend
Turn torso over leg and stretch forward
Place ball on floor in centre and roll forward
Roll back
Repeat

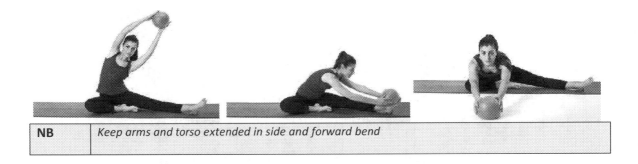

| NB | *Keep arms and torso extended in side and forward bend* |
|----|---------------------------------------------------------|

## Back and shoulder stretch

**Setup**    Kneeling with both hands resting on ball, arms straight
                Roll ball forward, feel as if you are pushing your body through your arms
                Roll ball backwards
                Repeat

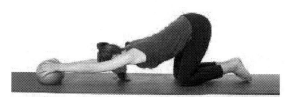

| **NB** | *Keep head lifted and in line with your body* | *Arms and torso stretched out* |
|--------|-----------------------------------------------|--------------------------------|

## Backward stretch

**Setup**    Lying supine, knees bent, ball between shoulder blades
                Support head with one hand, stretch other hand towards knees
                Extend body backwards, stretch arm overhead to touch floor at back
                Repeat

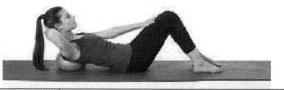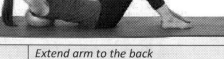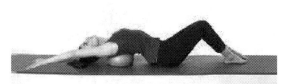

| **NB** | *Extend arm to the back* | *Feel the stretch in your arm, shoulders and back* |
|--------|--------------------------|----------------------------------------------------|

# Pilates Ring

## Spine twist

**Setup**     Standing, feet hip width apart, holding ring in front with both hands
                  Swing arms to side
                  Back to centre

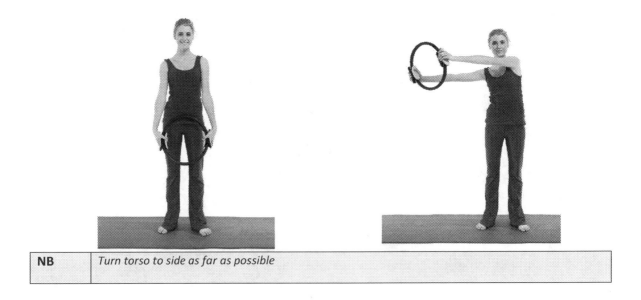

| NB | *Turn torso to side as far as possible* |
|----|------------------------------------------|

## Side bend

**Setup**     Standing, feet hip width apart, holding ring in front with both hands
                  Swing into side bend
                  Back to centre

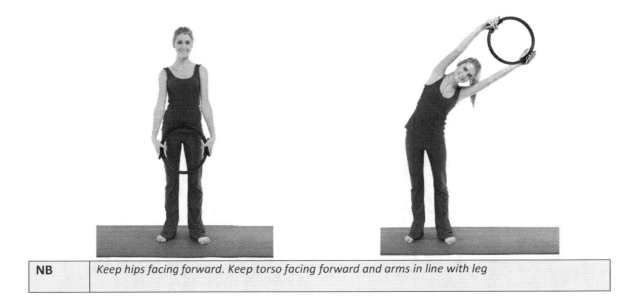

| NB | *Keep hips facing forward. Keep torso facing forward and arms in line with leg* |
|----|---------------------------------------------------------------------------------|

## Arm circles

**Setup**     Standing, feet hip width apart, holding ring with both hands
Swing arms in full circle
Repeat 10 x circle clockwise
Repeat 10 x circle anti-clockwise

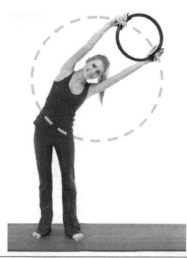

| **NB** | *Keep hips and torso facing forward* |
|--------|--------------------------------------|

## Shoulder Stretch

**Setup**     Standing, feet hip width apart, holding ring at back with both hands
Lift arms up
Lower arms
Repeat

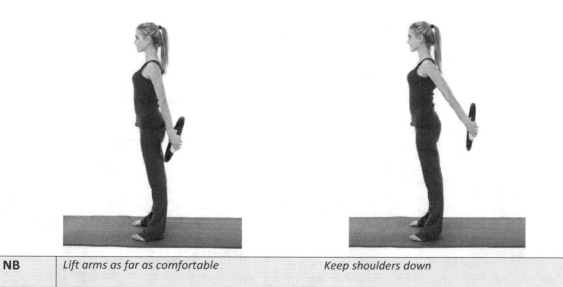

| **NB** | *Lift arms as far as comfortable* | *Keep shoulders down* |
|--------|-----------------------------------|------------------------|

## Pectoral stretch

**Setup**   Standing, feet hip width apart, holding ring at back with both hands
Lift arms at back, bend forward bringing arms over body
Lower arms
Repeat

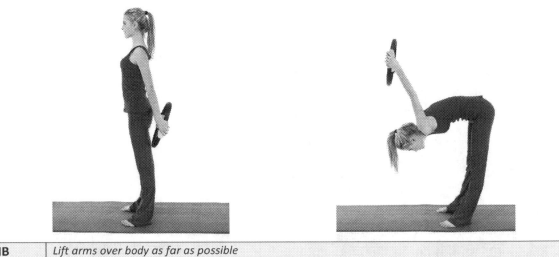

| NB | *Lift arms over body as far as possible* |
|----|------------------------------------------|

## Hamstring stretch

**Setup**   Lying supine, knees bent, one foot in ring, holding ring in both hands
Extend leg, pull ring towards chest
Repeat with other foot

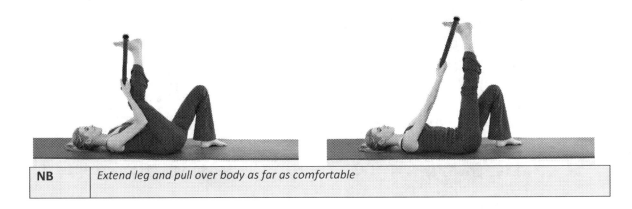

| NB | *Extend leg and pull over body as far as comfortable* |
|----|-------------------------------------------------------|

## Rocking

**Setup**    Lying prone, legs bent with feet hooked into ring, holding ring with both hands
                Lift torso and legs, hold onto ring
                Relax down to floor
                Repeat

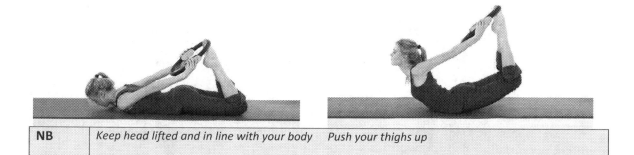

| NB | *Keep head lifted and in line with your body* | *Push your thighs up* |
|----|----|----|

## Back extensions

**Setup**    Lying prone, legs straight, holding ring with both hands
                Lift torso, push down on ring
                Relax down to floor
                Repeat

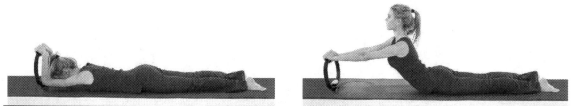

| NB | *Keep head in line with your body* | *Keep feet on floor* |
|----|----|----|

# *Thera Band*

## *Spine twist*

**Setup**     Standing, feet hip width apart, holding Thera band in front with both hands
              Lift arms and turn torso to face side, open arms to stretch band
              Back to front
              Repeat alternating sides

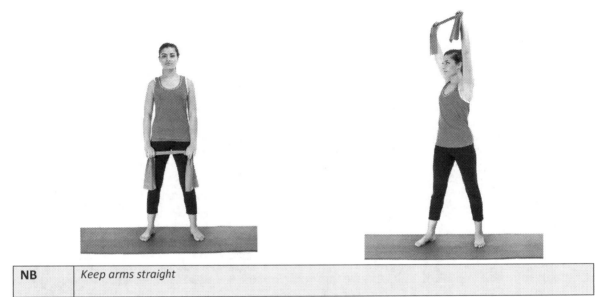

| NB | Keep arms straight |
|----|--------------------|

## *Shoulder stretch*

**Setup**     Standing, feet hip width apart, holding Thera band in front with both hands
              Swing arms upwards and lean backwards
              Lower arms
              Repeat

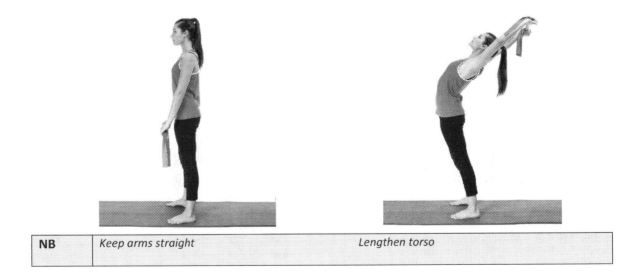

| NB | Keep arms straight | Lengthen torso |
|----|--------------------|----------------|

## Rotation with side bend

**Setup**     Standing, feet hip width apart, holding Thera band in front with both hands
              Turn torso to side, stretch arms overhead, pull into side bend
              Lower arms to front
              Repeat alternating sides

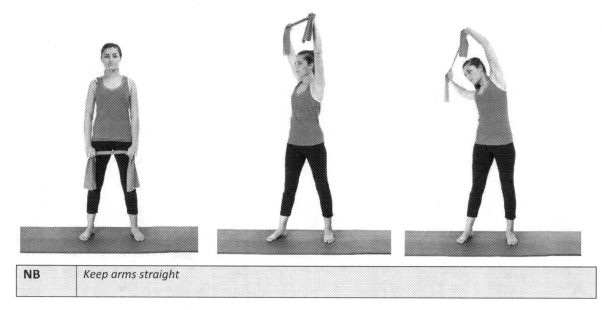

| NB | Keep arms straight |
|----|--------------------|

## Arms in full swing to back

**Setup**     Standing, feet hip width apart, holding Thera band in front with both hands
              Lift arms overhead to back
              Lift arms overhead to front
              Repeat

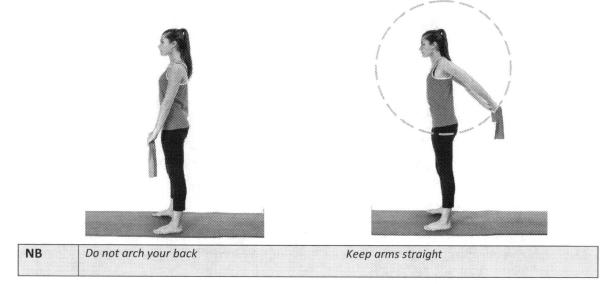

| NB | Do not arch your back | Keep arms straight |
|----|-----------------------|--------------------|

## Back arm lift

**Setup**    Standing, feet hip width apart, holding Thera band at back with both hands
Lift arms up, open arms to stretch band
Relax
Repeat

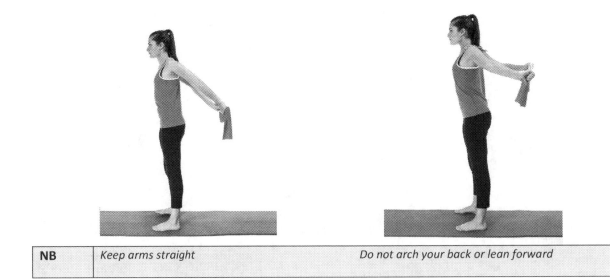

| NB | Keep arms straight | Do not arch your back or lean forward |
|----|--------------------|---------------------------------------|

## Side bend

**Setup**    Standing, feet hip width apart, holding Thera band in front with both hands
Lift arms into side bend, open arms to stretch band
Lower arms
Repeat

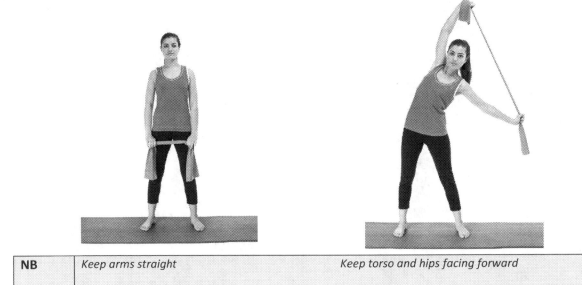

| NB | Keep arms straight | Keep torso and hips facing forward |
|----|--------------------|-----------------------------------|

## Full circle

**Setup**   Standing, feet wide apart, holding Thera band with both hands
Swing arms in full circle
Repeat 10 x clockwise
Repeat 10 x anti-clockwise

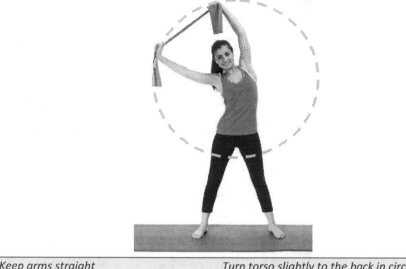

| NB | Keep arms straight | Turn torso slightly to the back in circles |
|---|---|---|

## Shoulder and arm Stretch

**Setup**   Standing, feet wide apart, holding Thera band at back at shoulder level
Stretch arms to back in line with shoulders
Bend arms back to shoulders
Repeat

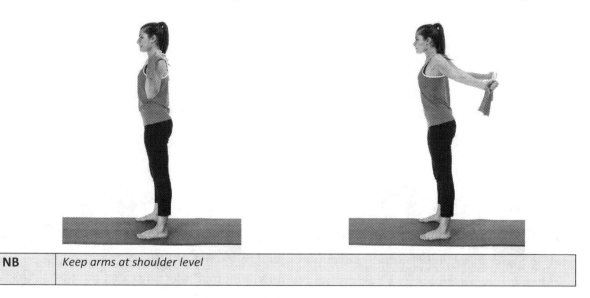

| NB | Keep arms at shoulder level | |
|---|---|---|

## Standing hamstring stretch

**Setup**   Standing with your back against the wall, one foot in Thera band
Stretch leg forward and lift up
Relax leg
Repeat

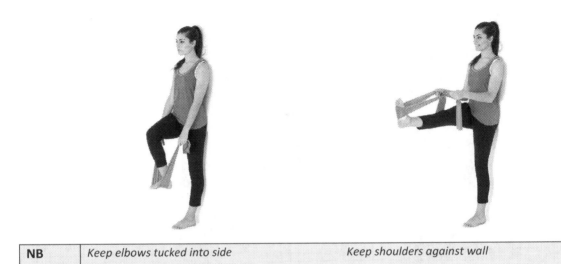

| NB | Keep elbows tucked into side | Keep shoulders against wall |
|----|------------------------------|------------------------------|

## Hamstring stretch

**Setup**   Lying supine, one knee bent and one foot in Thera band, elbows on floor
Lift leg and pull over body
Repeat with other foot

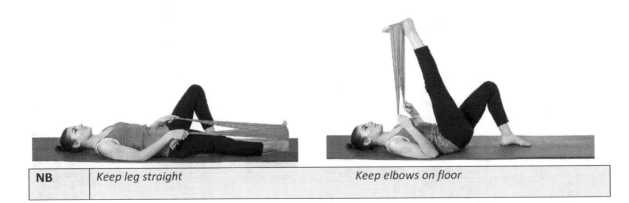

| NB | Keep leg straight | Keep elbows on floor |
|----|-------------------|----------------------|

## Double leg hamstring stretch

**Setup**    Lying supine, knees bent, both feet in Thera band, elbows on floor
                Stretch legs, pull toes down, push heels out
                Bend knees
                Repeat

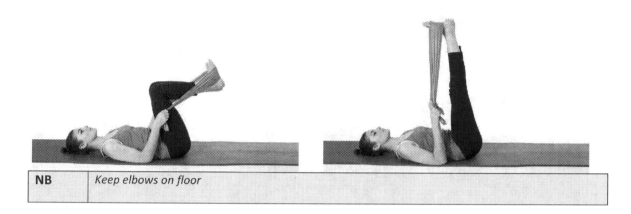

| NB | *Keep elbows on floor* |
|----|------------------------|

## Leg circles

**Setup**    Lying supine, one knee bent, one foot in Thera band, elbows on floor
                Lift leg up to 90 degrees, around to side in full circle
                Circle leg 5 x clockwise and 5 x anti clockwise
                Repeat with opposite leg

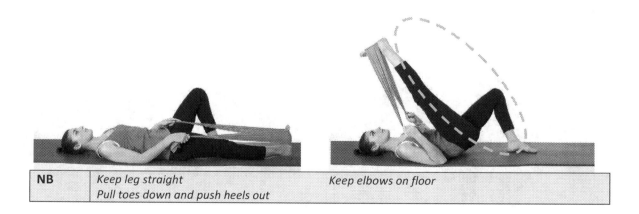

| NB | *Keep leg straight* | *Keep elbows on floor* |
|----|---------------------|------------------------|
|    | *Pull toes down and push heels out* | |

# Foam Roller

## Shoulder and back stretch

**Setup**     Sitting on bent legs, hands on roller
              Roll roller forwards, stretch out your torso as far as you can
              Feel as if you are pushing your body through your arms
              Roll roller backwards

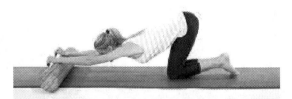

| NB | *Keep your arms straight* | *Elongate your torso* |
|----|---------------------------|-----------------------|

## Chest opener

**Setup**     Lying supine on roller, legs bent, both arms stretched upwards
              Open arms to touch floor on sides
              Lift arms upwards
              Repeat

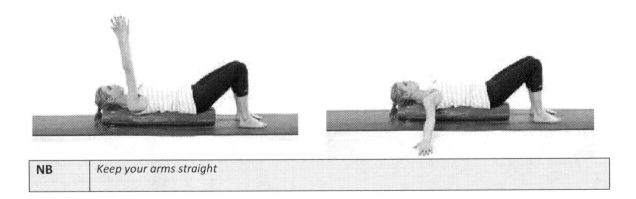

| NB | *Keep your arms straight* |
|----|---------------------------|

## Overhead stretch

**Setup**     Lying supine on roller, legs bent, both arms stretched upwards
Stretch arms overhead to touch floor
Lift arms upwards
Repeat

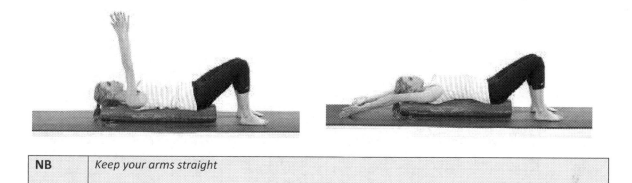

| NB | *Keep your arms straight* |
|---|---|

## Hip flexor stretch

**Setup**     Lying supine with roller under pelvis, legs bent, hands on roller
Pull one knee to towards  your chest
Slowly stretch leg out to touch floor
Repeat

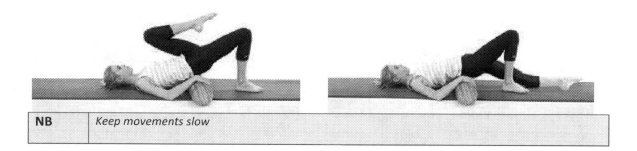

| NB | *Keep movements slow* |
|---|---|

## Leg extensions

**Setup**    Lying supine with roller under pelvis, holding one leg in both hands
                 Stretch  leg and flex foot
                 Relax
                 Repeat

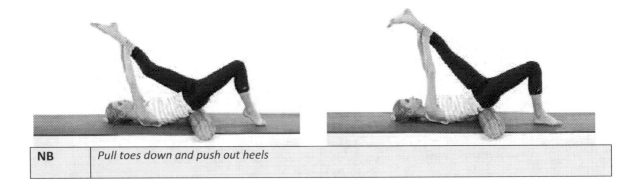

| NB | *Pull toes down and push out heels* |
|----|-------------------------------------|

## Hip opener with spine lift

**Setup**    Lying supine, one foot on roller, ankle on knee, arms on floor
                 Lift hips up
                 Relax
                 Repeat

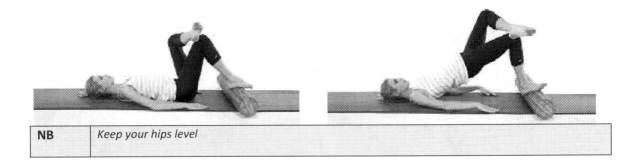

| NB | *Keep your hips level* |
|----|------------------------|

## Shoulder bridge

**Setup**      Lying supine, legs bent, feet on roller, palms on floor
                Lift hips, stretch one leg overhead
                Leg down to roller and lower hips
                Repeat

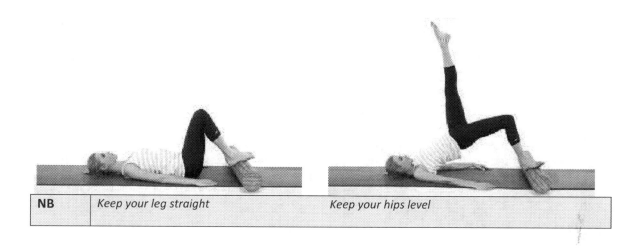

| NB | Keep your leg straight | Keep your hips level |
|----|------------------------|----------------------|

## Thigh stretch

**Setup**      Sitting on knees with hands on roller
                Lift your body, push hips out
                Sit down
                Repeat

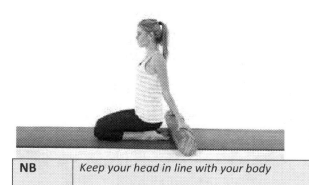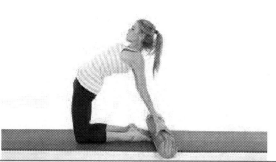

| NB | Keep your head in line with your body | Push up from your hips towards your shoulders |
|----|---------------------------------------|-----------------------------------------------|

## Back stretch

**Setup**    Lying prone, arms stretched forward, with wrists on roller
Lift torso, roll roller towards you
Roll roller away, lie down
Repeat

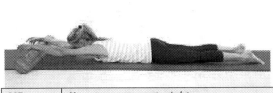
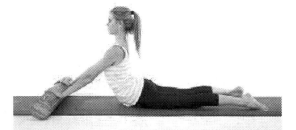

| NB | Keep your arms straight | Roll roller as close to body as possible |
|----|-------------------------|------------------------------------------|

## Hamstring stretch with legs open

**Setup**    Sitting with legs wide open, ankles on roller
Hold onto roller, pull yourself forwards
Relax
Repeat

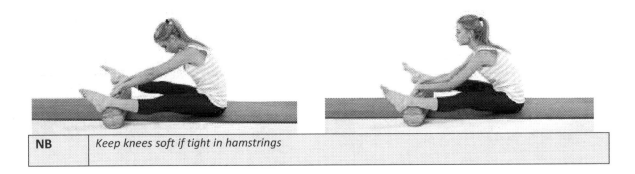

| NB | Keep knees soft if tight in hamstrings |
|----|----------------------------------------|

## Hamstring stretch with legs together

**Setup**     Sitting with legs straight, ankles on roller
               Hold onto roller, pull yourself forwards
               Relax
               Repeat

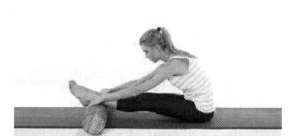

| NB | *Keep knees soft if tight in hamstrings* |
|----|------------------------------------------|

## Cross legged spine stretch

**Setup**     Sitting with legs folded, hands on roller
               Push roller forwards
               Pull roller backwards
               Fold legs the other way
               Repeat

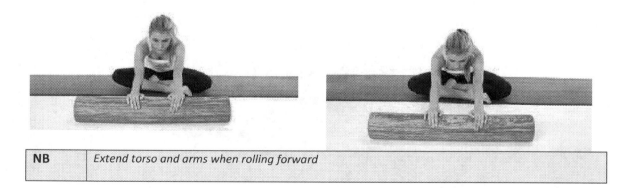

| NB | *Extend torso and arms when rolling forward* |
|----|----------------------------------------------|

# Foam Roller Body Massage

## Calve massage.

**Setup**    Sitting with calves resting on roller, hands at back for support
Roll your legs forwards and backwards on the roller

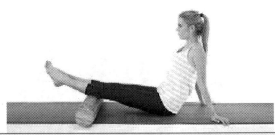

| NB | *Movements are small and only at your calves* |
|----|-----------------------------------------------|

## Upper leg massage

**Setup**    Lying on side with thigh resting on roller, one leg bent, elbow on floor for support
Roll your upper thigh up and down on the roller
Repeat other side

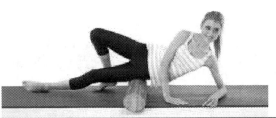

| NB | *Do not roll backwards* | *Stay on your side with the roller at your thigh* |
|----|-------------------------|---------------------------------------------------|

## Side massage

**Setup**    Lying on side with roller at your hip, one leg bent, elbow on floor for support
Roll up and down on the roller from hip up towards your arm
Repeat other side

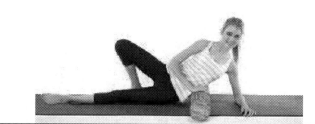

| NB | *Keep movements small* |
|----|------------------------|

## Thigh massage

**Setup**    Lying prone with thighs resting on roller, elbows on floor for support
Roll your body forwards and backwards on the roller

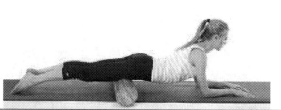

| NB | *Stay on your elbows* | *Don't sink in your lower back* |
|----|-----------------------|---------------------------------|

## Back massage

**Setup**    Lying prone with roller at lower back, both legs bent for support
Roll up and down on the roller

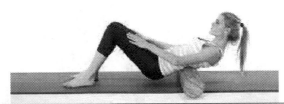

| NB | *Roll from lower back up towards your shoulders* |
|----|---------------------------------------------------|

## Relaxation

**Setup**    Lying with legs bent on either side of roller, head resting on roller
Relax

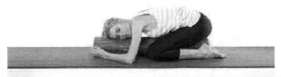

| NB | *Close your eyes and relax* |
|----|------------------------------|

# *The Pole*

## *Overhead reach*

**Setup**      Standing, feet wide apart, holding pole in front with both hands
Lift arms up and bend backwards
Arms to front
Repeat

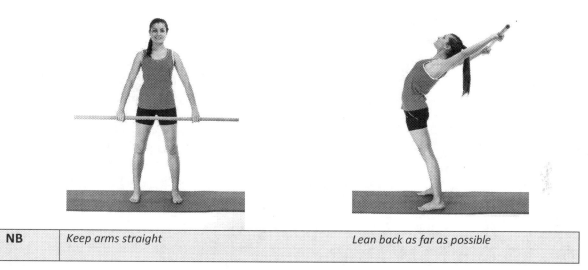

| **NB** | *Keep arms straight* | *Lean back as far as possible* |
|--------|----------------------|--------------------------------|

## *Side bend*

**Setup**      Standing, feet wide apart, holding pole in front with both hands
Swing arms up and into side bend
Back to front
Repeat

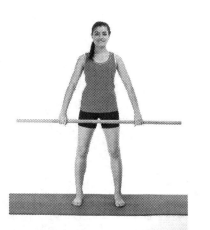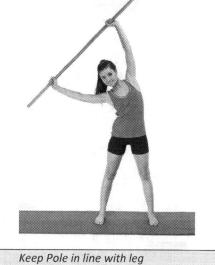

| **NB** | *Keep arms straight and torso facing forward* | *Keep Pole in line with leg* |
|--------|------------------------------------------------|------------------------------|

## Spine twist

**Setup**     Standing, feet wide apart, pole resting on shoulders, arms straight in T position
              Turn torso to face side
              Back to front
              Repeat

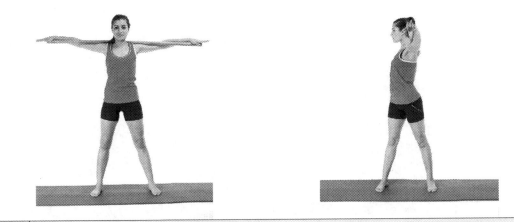

| NB | *Keep back straight and shoulders down* |
|----|------------------------------------------|

## Side tilt

**Setup**     Standing, feet wide apart, pole resting on shoulders, arms straight in T position
              Tilt into side bend
              Back to front
              Repeat

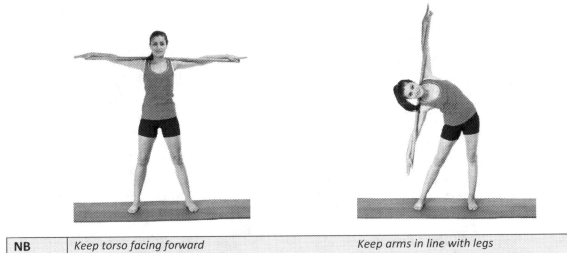

| NB | *Keep torso facing forward* | *Keep arms in line with legs* |
|----|-----------------------------|-------------------------------|

## Hamstring stretch

**Setup**    Sitting with pole behind bent leg, hands holding pole
Stretch leg
Bend leg
Repeat

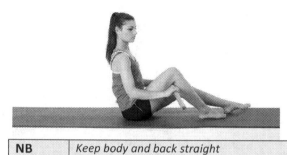 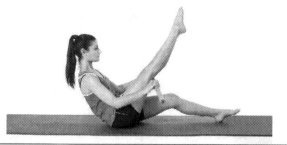

| NB | Keep body and back straight | Keep shoulders down |
|----|------------------------------|---------------------|

## Full stretch

**Setup**    Lying supine, legs straight, pole resting on thighs
Lift arms overhead to touch floor at back
Lift arms back to start position
Repeat

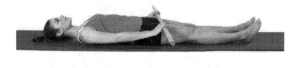 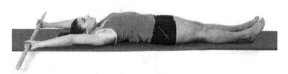

| NB | Feel overall stretch throughout your body | Stretch from your arms right down to your toes |
|----|--------------------------------------------|-------------------------------------------------|

## Side stretch with bent legs

**Setup**    Sitting with both legs bent to one side, arms stretched upwards
Swing pole into side bend over legs
Back to start position
Repeat

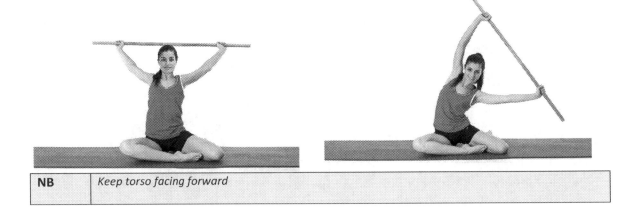

| NB | *Keep torso facing forward* |
|----|------------------------------|

## Side bend with straight leg

**Setup**    Sitting, one leg folded in, other leg stretched to side
Stretch into side bend, hold
Turn torso and stretch forward over leg
Back to start position
Repeat

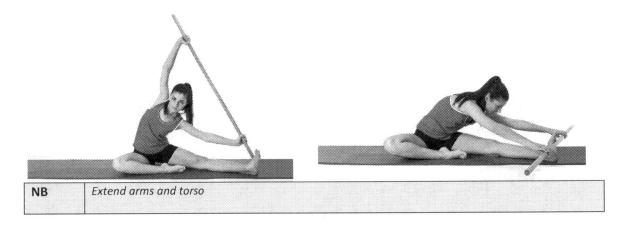

| NB | *Extend arms and torso* |
|----|--------------------------|

## Forward bend

**Setup**    Sitting upright with legs together, holding pole over feet
Pull into forward bend
Relax
Repeat

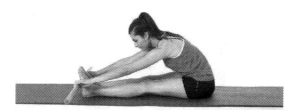

| NB | *Keep back straight and extend from hips* |
|----|-------------------------------------------|

## Hamstring stretch

**Setup**    Lying supine, one leg bent on floor, other leg straight, pole behind leg
Lift shoulders and stretch leg
Relax
Repeat

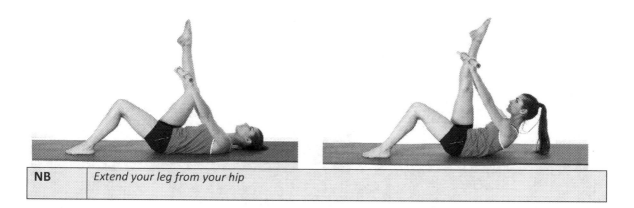

| NB | *Extend your leg from your hip* |
|----|----------------------------------|

## Arm and back stretch

**Setup**    Lying prone, holding pole at back with both hands
              Lift arms up
              Relax
              Repeat

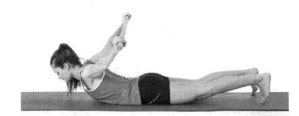

| NB | *Keep head in line with shoulders* |
|----|-----------------------------------|

## Partner stretch

**Setup**    Lying prone, holding pole at back with both hands
              Partner standing over you with feet holding your hips tight
              Partner lifts pole with both hands
              Relax
              Repeat

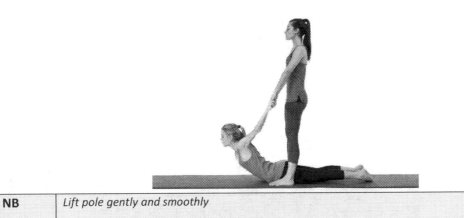

| NB | *Lift pole gently and smoothly* |
|----|--------------------------------|

# *Relaxation*

There is nothing more rewarding than relaxing after a strenuous workout. Have some soft music playing in the background.

Take a deep breath in and as you exhale, feel the tension flowing out of your body. Concentrate on your breathing and listen to the music. Do not let your mind wander. Relax your feet and legs, your hands, your arms, your stomach muscles, your chest, your neck and your facial muscles. Your body feels warm and heavy.

Try the following postures:

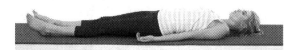

Lying supine, arms at your sides, palms facing upwards

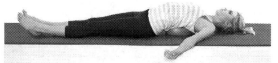

Lying supine with a deflated small ball between your shoulder blades, arms at your sides, palms facing upwards

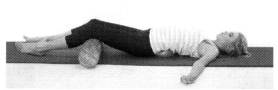

Lying supine with a foam roller under your knees and a deflated small ball under your lower back, arms at your sides, palms facing upwards

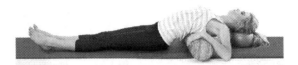

Lying supine with a roller under your shoulder blades
and a deflated small ball or cushion under your head

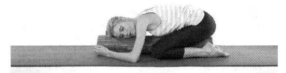

Lying prone with legs bent on either side of a foam roller, head resting on roller

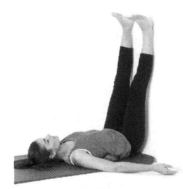

Lying with your legs and buttocks against a wall and a deflated small ball, towel
or bean bag under your pelvis, arms at your sides, palms facing upwards
*NB Your buttocks and legs must be against the wall*